LESSONS FROM THE SKY

LIFE FLIGHT RESCUES AND THE

FIGHT FOR CHILD SAFETY

David M Kaniecki DNP

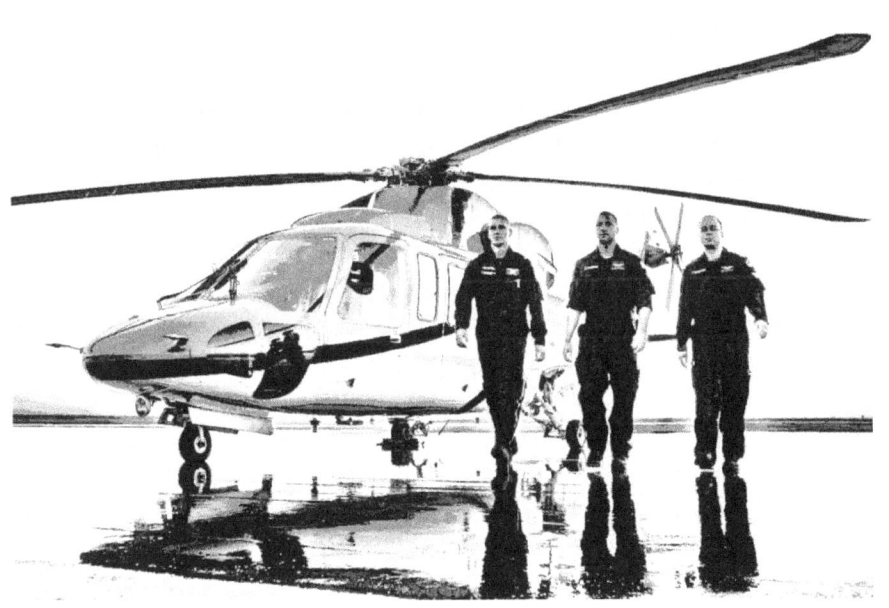

ISBN: 979-8-218-52179-0

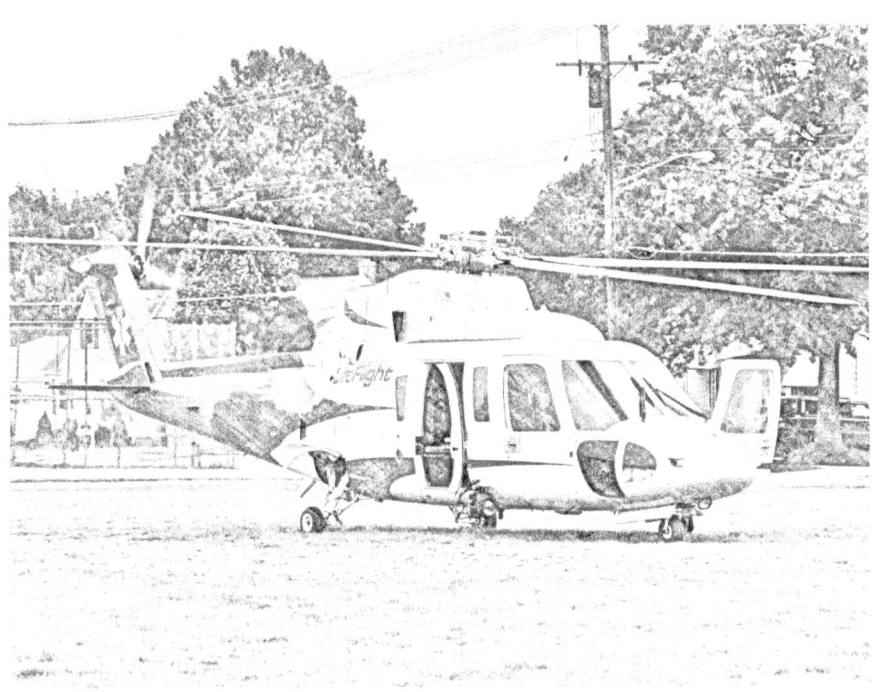

ABOUT THIS BOOK

Each year, over half a million Americans find themselves in need of urgent air medical transport. As a flight nurse, flight nurse practitioner, and critical care transport educator, I've seen many horrible accidents. The incidents that involve children are the ones that create the most heartbreaking memories. The sudden occurrence of an accident or illness can completely disrupt a child's life, causing families to feel overwhelmed by fear and uncertainty. My experiences and the stories shared by my colleagues serve as a stark reminder of life's fragility, particularly for our youngest patients.

This book speaks directly to parents, grandparents, and anyone who cares for children. Through the experiences of children who have faced emergencies, I aim to highlight the potential risks in our everyday surroundings. My goal is to raise awareness of these hazards and inspire you to act, creating safer spaces for our children to grow and thrive.

These narratives offer a window into the challenges faced by both young children and their families during times of crisis. You will gain a deeper understanding of the hidden risks that can threaten children's well-being and the vital role of

Emergency Medical Services (EMS) in delivering life-saving care.

Each story unfolds with a detailed account of the events leading up to the emergency, from the child's initial symptoms or injury to the rapid response of medical professionals. The journey from the frantic 911 call to the Life Flight helicopter at the hospital is described, underscoring the urgency and critical nature of these situations. Each story concludes with clear *'Take Home Points'* highlighting key lessons and practical steps to avoid similar incidents in the future.

While patient names and specific details have been changed to protect privacy, the essence of each story remains unchanged. I am confident that these real-life accounts will inform and empower you to take proactive measures to prevent accidents and be better prepared for emergencies.

My greatest hope is that by reading these stories of both heartbreak and hope, you will be inspired to create a safer world for the children you love. After all, they are our future, and their well-being is our most sacred responsibility.

My life's work has been dedicated to caring for the injured and educating others in the critical care transport field. However, I believe that preventing accidents is just as crucial as treating them.

I view this book as my contribution to ensuring a safe future for our children. By sharing these stories, I hope to empower you with knowledge and inspire you to take proactive measures to protect the young lives in your care. I sincerely hope that this book will prevent others, particularly children, from experiencing accident-related trauma.

I acknowledge that readers of this book come from diverse backgrounds and may have varying perspectives on the safety recommendations provided. The decision to implement these recommendations is a personal one. Parenting is a challenging task that requires balancing the safety of children with their development as individuals. Recognizing that each person may have different views on what constitutes optimal parenting, my goal is not to prescribe specific parenting methods but to raise awareness of potential safety hazards that might be easily overlooked.

Once again, this book includes narratives of children who have encountered unfortunate circumstances. There are those who have achieved remarkable recoveries, while others have suffered permanent disability or even death. Sensitive readers should consider this before proceeding. Through these stories, we remember, we learn, and we safeguard our children's future.

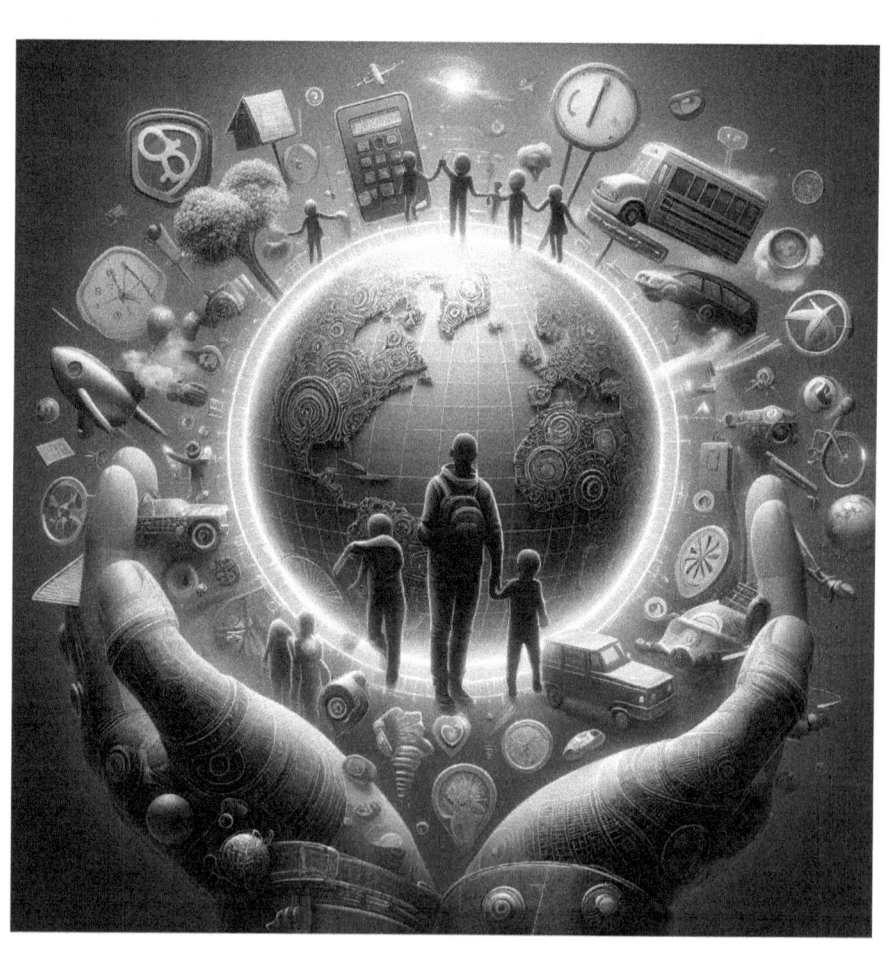

DISCLAIMER

An Advanced Practice Nurse Practitioner with a Doctor of Nursing Practice Degree authored this book. The author is not a physician and does not claim expertise in pediatric safety. This book is for informational purposes only, and the recommendations are derived from information that is openly accessible. Readers should conduct their own research and consult qualified professionals for specific concerns or decisions related to their child's safety. The author and publisher are not liable for any accidents or damages. Although we trust that the information is correct and logical, it's important to remember that even apparent details can be missed.

We aim to emphasize to readers the importance of recognizing potential risks and taking preventive actions, urging them to prioritize safety and alertness in their daily routines. For further information on child safety and accident prevention, consider consulting the following top websites and organizations:

Safe Kids Worldwide: www.safekids.org - A global organization dedicated to preventing childhood injuries, with information on a wide range of topics like car seat safety, fire safety, and sports safety.

Children's Safety Network: www.childrenssafetynetwork.org - Focuses on preventing injuries and violence, with resources for parents, professionals, and communities.

HealthyChildren.org: www.healthychildren.org/English/safety-prevention - From the American Academy of Pediatrics, this site offers comprehensive information on safety topics from birth to young adulthood.

CONTENTS

To my four wonderful children,

This book is a collection of the stories that have shaped my approach to parenting, directly affecting you. There were countless mornings when I would come home from work, lie down beside you as you slept, and thank God for your safety. From the moment you entered my life, I have made it my priority to ensure your well-being. Yet, I have always strived to balance your safety with the joy of childhood, allowing you to explore, jump, and play freely. My love for you is boundless, and I cherish every moment we share.

With all my heart,

Dad

A RIPPLE OF HOPE

In the small, quiet town of Willowbrook, the evening sun cast a warm glow on the white picket fences and neatly trimmed lawns. The neighborhood kids played together in the park, their laughter echoing through the streets. Life seemed perfect in this idyllic community.

In one of the charming houses on Maple Street, Emily Thompson was busy preparing dinner for her family. She hummed along to her favorite song on the radio as she chopped vegetables for a savory stew. It had been a long day, and Emily couldn't wait for her husband, Jack, to return home from work so they could enjoy a meal together with their two children, five-year-old Sarah and six-month-old Noah.

As Emily glanced at the clock, she realized it was nearly time for Noah's bath. Wanting to get a head start before Jack arrived, she quickly filled the bathtub with warm water, adding a few drops of lavender-scented baby wash. She then fetched Noah from his crib, where he cooed and giggled at her lovingly.

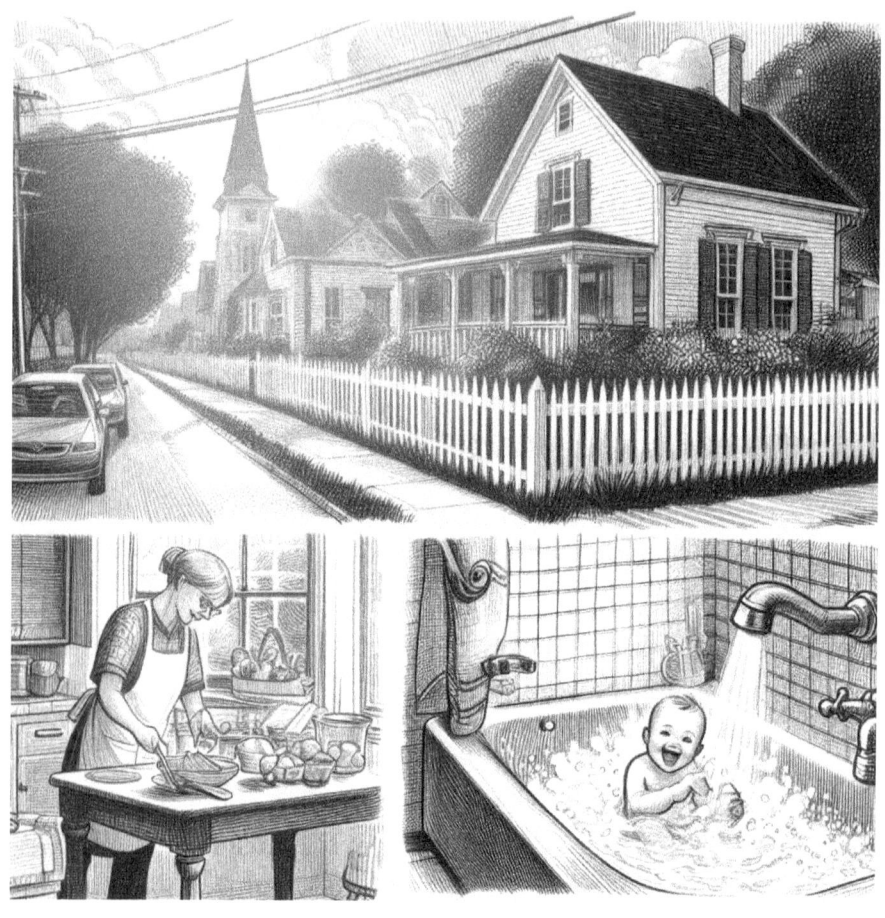

Emily gently lowered Noah into the tub, making sure the water was just the right temperature. He splashed happily as she washed him, his big blue eyes sparkling with delight. Emily couldn't resist smiling at her baby boy, filled with gratitude for the beautiful family she had been blessed with.

Suddenly, the phone rang in the living room, startling Emily. She hesitated for a moment, unsure whether to leave Noah unattended in the bathtub. But the persistent ringing convinced her it might be an important call. "It will only take a second," she thought, as she carefully placed a soft towel under Noah's head to support him.

Emily rushed to the living room, her heart pounding as she picked up the phone. It was Jack, calling to let her know he was stuck in traffic and would be home later than expected. As they spoke, Emily's concern grew, her mind racing with thoughts of how she could manage dinner, bath time, and bedtime alone.

During their conversation, a sudden silence fell upon the house, followed by a faint splash from the bathroom. Panic washed over Emily as she dropped the phone and sprinted back to the bathtub, fearing the worst.

To her horror, she found Noah submerged under the water, his tiny body limp and lifeless. Emily's heart shattered into a thousand pieces as she pulled him out of the tub, tears streaming down her face. She called 911 and desperately tried to revive him, performing CPR while pleading for him to wake up.

Meanwhile, the Emergency Medical Services (EMS) team had just finished a patient transport when they got the dreaded call to respond to an emergency involving a 6-month-old baby. Their hearts sank as they drove towards the address, silently praying that it would not be too late.

When they arrived, Emily was in tears and frantic with worry about her beloved child. The EMS crew quickly took charge of the situation, determined to do everything within their power to save this tiny life - but all without success until one of them detected a faint pulse! A miracle! Everyone sighed with relief as they carefully placed the baby onto a stretcher and transported him to the hospital where he could receive specialist care.

Upon arrival at the hospital, the tiny patient remained unresponsive despite passionate efforts made to rouse him.

With the child struggling to breathe on his own, the medical team moved quickly and purposefully, placing a breathing tube, and providing vital ventilator support. Tears welled up in the eyes of every onlooker and the little one's parents held onto each other tightly as the team worked to keep him alive. Due to the hospital's limited resources, the baby would need to be transferred to a higher level of care via air medical transport, heroically fighting to stay alive with every moment that passed.

As the helicopter blades sliced through the air, the Life Flight team sprang into action. The sun dipped below the horizon, painting the sky in hues of orange and pink, but the beauty of the scene was lost on Michelle, the flight nurse. Her thoughts were consumed by the mission at hand: saving the life of a six-month-old baby who had nearly drowned.

Michelle understood the importance of every second in situations like these. She couldn't help but think about what the baby's parents must be going through: the terror, the guilt, and the overwhelming sense of helplessness as they waited for help to arrive. It was a feeling she knew all too well from her own experiences.

In the confined space of the helicopter, Michelle meticulously prepared the necessary equipment, making sure everything was ready for the infant's arrival. She thought about the countless hours spent training and the numerous lives she had helped save during her career. But this time felt different. This time, it was personal.

Years ago, her own nephew had faced a similar situation – an accident in the bathtub that left him fighting for his life. The memory of that day was etched into her mind, and she knew she couldn't let history repeat itself. She silently vowed to do everything in her power to save this little life.

As the helicopter descended upon the small hospital, Michelle's heart pounded in her chest. She inhaled slowly to prepare herself for what was ahead. Once the crew landed, they wasted no time and made their way inside the hospital.

As the doors opened, she caught sight of the frantic parents, their eyes filled with fear and hope. In that moment, Michelle knew she was not just a flight nurse; she was a lifeline for this family in their darkest hour.

The baby was swiftly placed on the monitoring equipment and ventilator for transportation, and then loaded onto the helicopter. Michelle skillfully and purposefully used her hands to provide care, while her mind rapidly considered various scenarios and potential outcomes. She knew that there was no room for error, and she refused to let this child slip away.

Michelle was filled with determination as the helicopter flew to the large academic hospital. Saving countless lives before, she would do whatever it took to save this little one. Michelle knew in that fragile balance between life and death that she had to do whatever it took to give Noah the best chance of making a comeback.

In Noah's case, every second counted. Thanks to Michelle's unwavering efforts, Baby Noah was safely transported to a higher level of medical care, where he received the best chance at recovery.

The medical team ran tests and observed Noah for hours…then days. Heartbreakingly, it was concluded that the oxygen deprivation during the drowning incident resulted in neurological damage. As everyone's heart broke into pieces, it was hard to fathom how a soul so young and innocent could have suffered so much. But in the darkest of moments, sometimes miracles happen. And indeed, on day three, something extraordinary happened – Baby Noah opened his eyes. Though unable to move because of the brain damage sustained during the incident, there was now hope for his future.

Michelle's swift actions and the medical team's expertise gave Baby Noah another chance at life. Even though he may never fully recover from what happened that fateful day, his story is a reminder that hope and miracles can be found even in the bleakest of moments.

Take Home Points

A 6-month-old baby can drown in a bathtub because of several factors:

Lack of supervision: Babies at this age cannot sit up independently and can easily slip or tip over in the water. If left unattended, even for a moment, they can become submerged and unable to lift their head above water.

Shallow water: It doesn't take much water for a baby to drown. As little as 2 inches (5 centimeters) of water can pose a risk if a baby's face is submerged.

Inexperience: Babies cannot hold their breath and do not have the physical strength to move themselves out of a dangerous situation.

Reflexes: When a baby's face comes in contact with water, it may trigger an involuntary reflex called the "gasp reflex," causing the baby to inhale water involuntarily.

To prevent such tragic incidents, it's crucial to supervise babies closely during bath time and never leave them unattended, even for a brief period. By using safety equipment such as non-slip bathmats and baby bath seats, the risks of inadvertent slipping and accidental submersion can be reduced.

SHATTERED DREAMS

The sun was just beginning to rise, casting a warm golden glow over the quaint suburban neighborhood. Birds sang their morning melodies, and the air was crisp and invigorating. It was the perfect time for a morning jog.

Melanie, a young mother in her early thirties, laced up her running shoes and secured her six-month-old baby, Abigail, into the jogging stroller. As she stepped out of the house, she blew a kiss to her husband, Jake, who was busy preparing breakfast in the kitchen. He smiled back at her and waved goodbye, knowing that these morning jogs were an essential part of Melanie's routine.

As Melanie jogged along the tree-lined streets, she felt a sense of peace and contentment. The rhythmic sound of her footsteps and the gentle motion of the stroller lulled Abigail into a peaceful slumber. Melanie cherished these moments, where it was just her, her baby, and the open road.

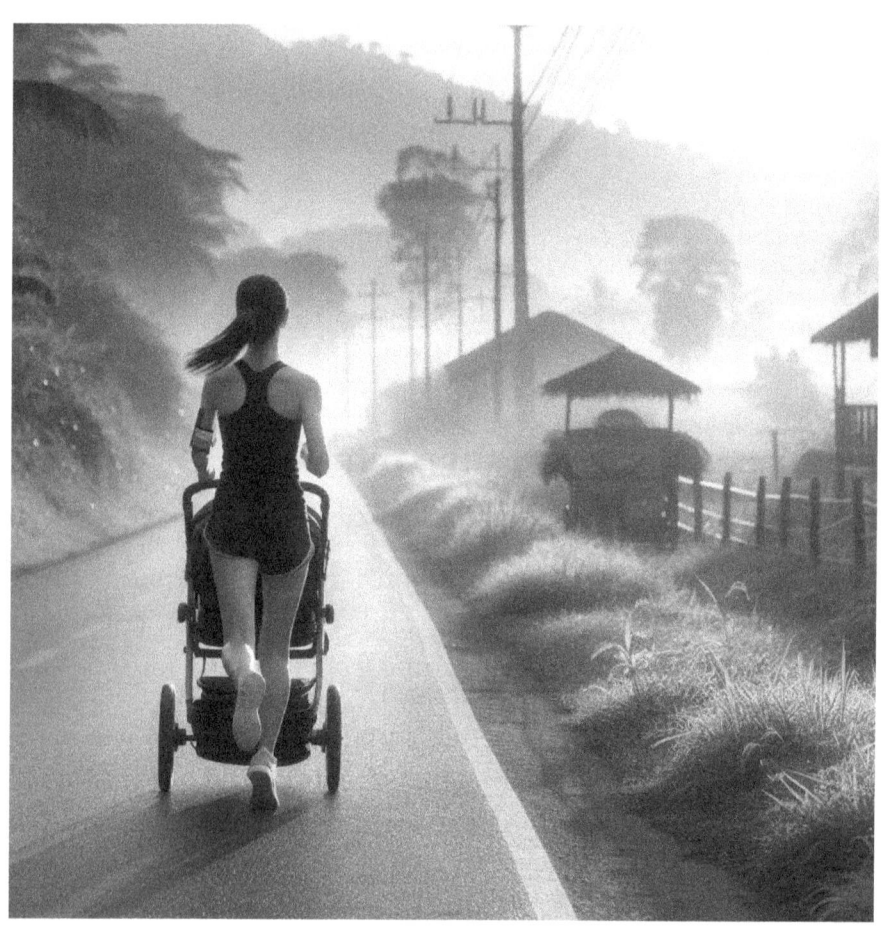

A few blocks away, a young teenager named Tyler was running late for school. His phone buzzed incessantly with texts from his friends, and he couldn't resist the temptation to respond as he drove. His eyes darted between the road and his phone screen, completely oblivious to the potential danger he posed.

As Melanie rounded a corner, she noticed the approaching car but assumed the driver would slow down. She continued jogging, not realizing that Tyler's attention was focused on his phone instead of the road. In a split second, the unthinkable happened. Tyler's car veered off the road, striking

Melanie and the jogging stroller with a sickening crash. The force of the impact launched Melanie and Abigail into the air, their fates uncertain.

The sound of sirens filled the air as Emergency Medical Services (EMS) arrived at the scene. Paramedics quickly assessed the situation, realizing that both Melanie and Abigail required immediate medical attention. Two air medical helicopters were dispatched, one for each patient. In order to avoid overloading one Trauma Center with two patients, Melanie and Abigail would be flown to separate places.

The scene was illuminated by the sun as the first helicopter landed. The flight team was summoned to transport Melanie to the nearest hospital following the car accident caused by a texting driver.

As they carefully loaded Melanie into the helicopter, the flight nurses discussed how tragic this accident was and hoped that she would be ok. They all were experienced professionals, yet their hearts still ached for Melanie's family waiting at home for news of their loved one's condition.

Once everyone was on board and ready to go, they took off toward their destination. As they flew through the blue sky, they looked down below at all of the hustle and bustle of life going on without them, knowing what had happened just moments before with Melanie. A solemn silence filled up inside of them as thoughts raced through each flight nurse's mind about how something like this could have happened so quickly to someone who simply wanted nothing more than to spend time with her family during such a beautiful morning.

It seemed like no time passed until finally reaching their destination; it felt like an eternity for those onboard, but it gave them peace knowing that soon enough Melanie would get proper medical treatment where maybe even miracles could happen if there was any hope left in this situation. After landing they rushed out of the helicopter with urgency, transferring Melanie into an ambulance and then on to the nearby Trauma Center.

The second helicopter carrying Nurse Emma, Nurse Will, and their precious cargo, six-month-old Abigail took off toward the Trauma Center. The entire flight there was filled with tension as every minute felt like an eternity for Emma and Will. All that mattered now was getting Baby Abigail safely to the hospital so she could be given medical attention. In between bouts of anxiousness, both nurses marveled at how beautiful it looked from up above – seeing everything from such great heights made them realize just how small their problems were in comparison to those of the world around them.

When they finally arrived at the Trauma Center—though it felt like hours, it had only been fifteen minutes—the two nurses swiftly exited the aircraft with Baby Abigail. They moved with urgency and precision into the emergency department, promptly handing over their patient. While doing so, they provided a thorough briefing on all events leading up to her arrival, ensuring seamless communication and immediate care without any delays or misunderstandings.

After watching helplessly as doctors pulled the curtains closed in the room for further examination of Baby Abigail, Nurses Emma and Will shared a look – one full of sadness yet also hope that this tiny life would make it through despite all odds being stacked against her. It was then that they realized just how much this experience meant not only for Abigail but also themselves; it wasn't about heroism or bravery but simply doing what you can do to help no matter who or where you are.

At the Trauma Center, doctors and nurses sprang into action, desperately trying to save Melanie's life. They worked tirelessly, employing every available resource and technique. Despite their relentless efforts, her traumatic injuries were too severe. Melanie passed away, surrounded by a dedicated team of medical professionals who had fought valiantly to keep her alive. Their faces reflected the sorrow of losing a patient they had strived so hard to save.

Meanwhile, at the other Trauma Center, Baby Abigail was in critical condition but showing promising signs of improvement. The dedicated medical team worked tirelessly, providing round-the-clock care to ensure her survival. They closely monitored her progress, adjusting treatments as needed and celebrating each small victory. Their unwavering commitment and attention to detail gave hope that Abigail would continue to recover.

When Jake received the devastating news about Melanie's death, his world came crashing down. The love of his life, his partner, and the mother of his child was gone. As he grappled with his grief, he knew he needed to stay strong for Abigail, who was still fighting for her life.

Days turned into weeks, and Abigail slowly began to recover. The medical team marveled at her resilience, and it wasn't long before she was discharged from the hospital. As Jake carried his baby girl out of the hospital and into their new reality, he vowed to honor Melanie's memory by being the best father he could be.

Over the years, Jake poured his heart and soul into raising Abigail. He taught her about the importance of kindness, compassion, and perseverance – values that Melanie had held dear. As Abigail grew older, he shared stories of her mother's life, ensuring that she would always know how much Melanie loved her.

Through the heartache and pain, Jake found solace in his role as a single father. He watched with pride as Abigail blossomed into a strong, intelligent, and compassionate young woman – a testament to the love and dedication he had poured into her upbringing.

On the day Abigail graduated from high school, Jake stood in the audience with tears in his eyes. As she walked across the stage to accept her diploma, he knew that Melanie would be proud of the person their daughter had become.

Texting and driving is a dangerous and potentially life-threatening behavior that should be avoided at all costs. There are several reasons why it is essential not to text while driving:

Distracted driving: Texting diverts a driver's attention from the primary task of driving, as it requires visual, manual, and cognitive focus. This distraction increases the risk of accidents, putting the driver, passengers, and other road users in danger.

Slower reaction time: When drivers are engaged in texting, their reaction times are significantly slower. They may not be able to react quickly enough to avoid collisions or respond to sudden changes in traffic conditions, such as a car stopping abruptly in front of them.

Impaired judgment: Texting while driving can impair a driver's ability to make sound decisions, as their focus is divided between the conversation and the road. This can lead to poor judgment calls, such as failing to yield the right of way or misjudging the speed of other vehicles.

Increased crash risk: Studies have shown that texting while driving increases the risk of a crash by 23 times compared to undistracted driving. This risk is even higher for inexperienced drivers, such as teenagers.

Legal consequences: Many countries and states have enacted laws prohibiting texting while driving, with penalties ranging from fines to license suspension or even jail time. Engaging in this behavior could result in legal repercussions and increased insurance premiums.

Social responsibility: As members of society, we have a responsibility to keep ourselves and others safe. By choosing not to text and drive, we demonstrate our commitment to maintaining a safe environment on the road for everyone.

Instead of texting while driving, consider alternative solutions to stay connected:

- Use a hands-free device or voice-activated technology to send and receive messages.
- Pull over to a safe location before reading or responding to messages.
- Inform friends and family that you will not be available to text while driving and encourage them to do the same.

By understanding the dangers of texting and driving and adopting safer practices, we can work together to reduce the number of accidents and fatalities caused by this risky behavior.

Jogging with a stroller on the side of the road can be a dangerous activity for both the parent and the child. There are several reasons why this is not an ideal way to exercise, as well as safer alternatives to consider.

First, the proximity to traffic puts both the jogger and the child at risk. Cars may not always keep a safe distance from the side of the road, and there is the potential for accidents to occur, such as distracted drivers texting and driving. Additionally, poor visibility due to weather conditions or blind spots might make it difficult for drivers to see the jogger and stroller.

Second, uneven terrain and roadside debris can be hazardous. Potholes, cracks, and loose gravel can cause the stroller to become unstable, increasing the risk of accidents. Furthermore, broken glass, nails, or other sharp objects might puncture the stroller's tires or cause injuries to the jogger.

To ensure a safer jogging experience with a stroller, consider the following alternatives:

Choose dedicated paths: Choose jogging routes specifically designed for pedestrians, such as parks, trails, and sidewalks. These areas usually have smoother surfaces and are separated from traffic, reducing the risk of accidents.

Use a jogging stroller: Invest in a stroller specifically designed for jogging, which typically features larger, air-filled tires, and better suspension to handle uneven terrain. These strollers also have a hand brake for added control and safety.

Be visible: Wear brightly colored clothing and use reflective gear on both you and the stroller. This makes it easier for drivers to spot you, especially during early morning or evening jogs when visibility is low.

Run against traffic: If you must jog on the side of the road, face oncoming traffic so you can see approaching vehicles and react accordingly.

Stay alert: Avoid using headphones while jogging, as they can distract you from your surroundings. Instead, stay aware of the environment and potential hazards.

By taking these precautions and choosing safer alternatives, parents can still enjoy jogging with their child while minimizing the risks associated with running on the side of the road.

COLLISION OF INNOCENCE

In a small suburban town, there lived a six-year-old boy named Timmy. He had dark brown eyes and brown hair that seemed to bounce with every step he took. His laughter was infectious, and his curiosity knew no bounds. Timmy was the pride of his family, who adored him more than anything in the world.

One sunny afternoon, Timmy's father asked him to fetch the mail from their mailbox across the road. Though Timmy was young, he had done this task many times before, always under the watchful eye of his parents. But today, his father was preoccupied with an urgent phone call, and he underestimated the danger that lay ahead.

With a sense of excitement and responsibility, Timmy eagerly accepted the task. He stepped out of the house and took a deep breath, the fresh air filling his lungs. The road in front of their home seemed quiet.

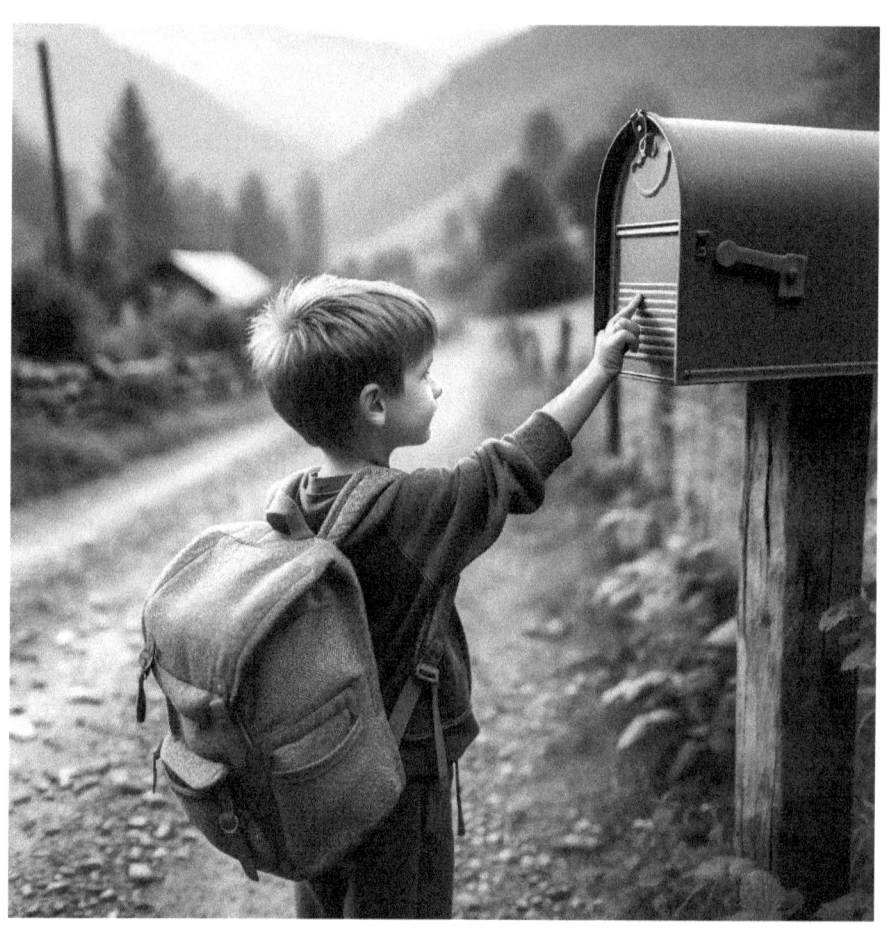

As Timmy approached the road, he remembered his father's advice: "Always look both ways and wait for the right moment to cross." So, he stood at the edge of the road, scanning the traffic for a safe gap. His small heart raced with anticipation, feeling a mix of fear and thrill.

A few moments later, Timmy spotted an opening in the traffic and believed it was his chance to cross. He took a deep breath and dashed across the road, his tiny legs pumping as fast as they could. However, just as he was about to reach the other side, a car appeared out of nowhere.

The driver, a young woman named Sarah, slammed on her brakes as soon as she saw Timmy, but it was too late. The car struck the little boy, sending him flying through the air and landing 40 feet away. The sound of the collision echoed through the air.

Timmy's father, still on the phone, heard the commotion and rushed outside to see his worst nightmare unfolding before his eyes. He dropped the phone, his heart shattering into a million pieces as he sprinted towards his son. Sarah, the driver, was also devastated, her face wet with tears as she exited her car to check on Timmy.

The entire neighborhood came together in those harrowing moments, with people calling for an ambulance and trying to provide comfort to Timmy's family. When the paramedics arrived, they quickly assessed Timmy's condition, finding him unconscious with multiple severe injuries.

With utmost care, they stabilized Timmy's head and neck, gently securing him onto a backboard and applying a neck brace. Every movement was deliberate, ensuring his spine remained protected. Once secured, Timmy was carefully lifted onto a stretcher and then into the ambulance. The doors slammed shut, and the ambulance sped away.

Sirens wailing, the ambulance carrying Timmy raced towards the nearest hospital. His parents, their faces etched with worry, headed there as well, their prayers a desperate plea for their son's survival. Recognizing the need for specialized care, the EMS team requested a Life Flight helicopter to meet their ambulance and transport Timmy directly to a Trauma Center.

Upon landing on the helipad of the small hospital, the air medical transport team hurriedly entered the emergency room (ER) with a clear objective: to stabilize and transfer young Timmy to the closest Trauma Center. Timmy's condition was rapidly worsening. His oxygen levels were dangerously low, and he was struggling to fill his tiny chest with enough air to survive.

The medical team quickly assessed the situation and determined that Timmy needed both a breathing tube and a chest tube to help him breathe. A chest tube is a thin, hollow tube which is carefully inserted between the ribs, into the space around the lungs. This allows air and fluid to drain, relieving pressure and helping the lungs to expand fully.

In the intense atmosphere of the ER, the emergency doctor skillfully inserted the chest and breathing tubes with the help of the Life Flight team. With each deliberate motion, a subtle shift could be seen in Timmy's breathing, his once-desperate gasps becoming slightly less labored.

Once Timmy was stable enough for transport, the Life Flight team carefully loaded him onto the helicopter, his tiny body swaddled in blankets and connected to numerous machines monitoring his vital signs. Timmy's mother, heart heavy with worry, boarded the helicopter alongside her son. Fear visible on her face, she tightly gripped Timmy's hand, praying for a miracle. The roar of the helicopter's engine filled the air as it lifted off, soaring high above the scenic landscape below.

The atmosphere was tense and focused inside the helicopter. The Life Flight crew closely monitored Timmy's condition, adjusting medications and life support equipment as needed to maintain his fragile stability. They exchanged urgent and short radio communication, their eyes never leaving the monitors displaying Timmy's heart rate, blood pressure, and oxygen levels.

The flight to the Trauma Center was fraught with anxiety. As the afternoon sun cast long shadows over the ground, the Life Flight team continued their tireless efforts to keep Timmy stable.

As the helicopter approached the city, the skyline's towering buildings came into view, signaling that they were nearing their destination. The Life Flight crew prepared for landing, double-checking Timmy's equipment to ensure a smooth transfer once they arrived at the Trauma Center.

Upon touching down on the Trauma Center's helipad, the Life Flight team wasted no time in rushing Timmy into the emergency department. Doctors and nurses stood ready, immediately taking over his care and whisking him away for further evaluation and treatment.

The doctors and nurses worked tirelessly, doing everything in their power to save Timmy. After hours of surgery and anxious waiting, the doctors emerged with solemn expressions.

Though they had managed to stabilize Timmy's condition, it was clear that the road to recovery would be long and uncertain. His mother was grateful for the medical team's efforts but feared that their lives would never be the same.

The weeks that followed were a blur of sterile hallways, hushed conversations, and the constant beeping of machines. Timmy endured countless tests, procedures, and surgeries, his small body bearing the weight of the accident's aftermath. His parents kept a constant vigil by his bedside, their faces etched with worry and exhaustion.

The hospital staff became like an extended family, offering support and encouragement amidst the uncertainty. It was a long, arduous journey, fraught with setbacks and moments of despair, but Timmy's fighting spirit, fueled by the love and prayers of those around him, never wavered.

After what felt like an eternity, the day finally arrived when Timmy was discharged from the hospital. Though his homecoming was filled with joy and relief, the journey was far from over. Months of intensive rehabilitation followed. With each small victory, whether it was taking his first steps or uttering his first words after the accident, his family's hearts swelled with pride and gratitude. Through it all, Timmy's spirit remained unbroken.

Timmy's infectious laughter returned to the neighborhood slowly over time. Every day, he showed improvement, his energy seemingly limitless, and the scars on his body serving as a testament to his incredible resilience. The accident permanently changed their lives and strengthened the community bond. Timmy, the brave little boy, triumphed over tragedy, serving as a beacon of hope for all.

Timmy celebrated his remarkable recovery surrounded by loved ones on a sunny afternoon about a year after the ordeal. The EMS crew, Life Flight team, and ER hospital staff who had helped stabilize Timmy prior to his transfer to the Trauma Center all joined, their faces filled with pride and gratitude. It was a heartwarming scene, showcasing dedication and collaboration that saved Timmy's life.

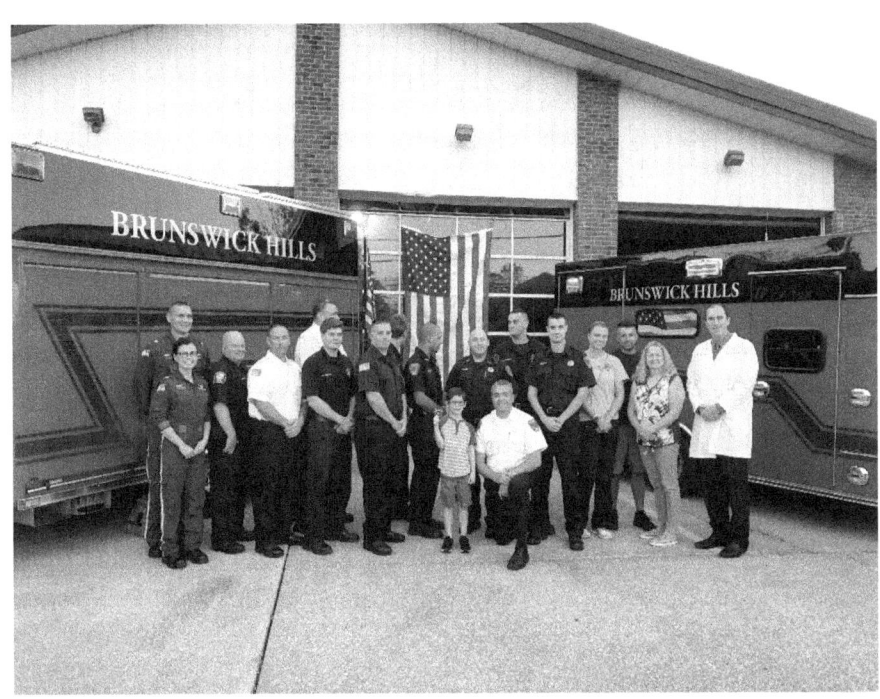

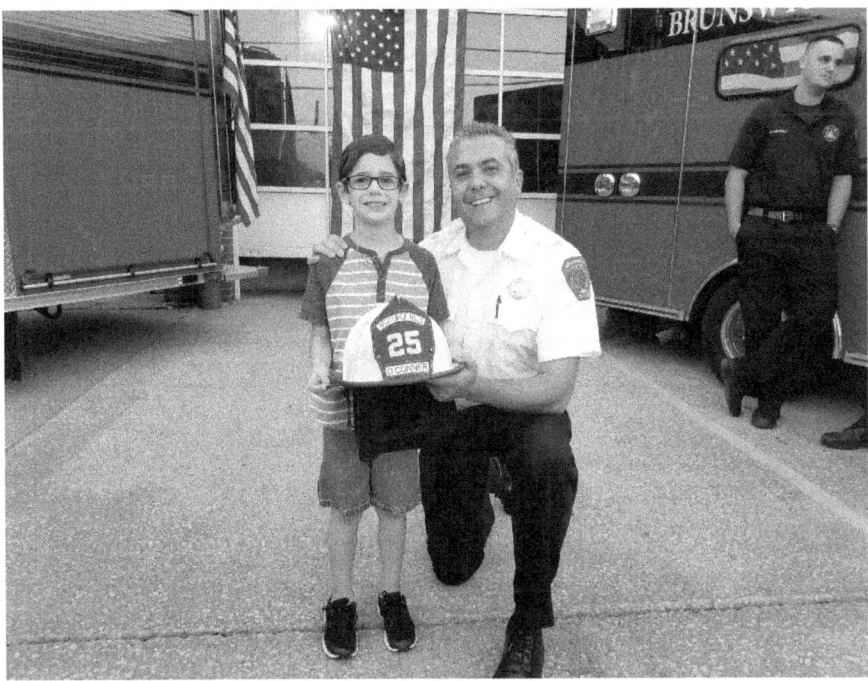

Take Home Points

Roads can be busy, fast-paced environments that pose significant risks for pedestrians, especially children. Allowing children to cross roads by themselves, without the proper education and maturity, can lead to catastrophic consequences such as severe injuries or even fatalities. It's difficult to pinpoint the exact age at which every child is ready to navigate roads alone, as it varies depending on individual development and the specific road conditions. Below, we discuss the various dangers associated with letting children navigate these high-speed roads on their own.

Lack of experience and judgement: Children have less experience and understanding of traffic rules compared to adults. They may not accurately gauge the speed and distance of oncoming vehicles, making it difficult for them to determine when it's safe to cross the road. Additionally, their decision-making skills are still developing, which means they might make impulsive choices that put them in harm's way.

Limited visibility: Young children are typically shorter than adults, which can make it difficult for drivers to spot them on the road. Moreover, children might be unable to see over obstacles like parked cars or bushes, hindering their ability to assess the situation properly. This limited visibility can lead to accidents as drivers may not have enough time to react when a child suddenly appears on the road.

Inattention and distractions: Children can be easily distracted by their surroundings or electronic devices, such as smartphones and tablets. This inattention can cause them to lose focus while crossing the road, increasing the likelihood of an accident. Furthermore, children are more prone to engaging in risky behavior like running across the road without looking or attempting to retrieve a dropped object from the road.

Driver behavior: Unfortunately, not all drivers follow the speed limits and traffic rules, and some may even be under the influence of alcohol or drugs. This reckless behavior puts all pedestrians at risk, but children are particularly vulnerable due to their small size and lack of experience. A child crossing the road by themselves is at the mercy of these irresponsible drivers.

High-speed traffic: Roads are designed for vehicles to travel at high speeds, making it extremely dangerous for pedestrians to cross. The faster a vehicle is moving, the less time a driver has to react to a child entering the roadway. Even if a child manages to gauge the speed of an oncoming car correctly, there's always the risk of a sudden lane change or a vehicle unexpectedly accelerating, which could lead to a tragic accident.

In conclusion, letting children cross roads by themselves can be a risky decision that puts their lives at risk. To ensure their safety, it's vital that parents and guardians educate their children about road safety rules and always accompany them when crossing busy roads. Additionally, advocating for safer pedestrian infrastructure like footbridges and implementing strict traffic laws can help reduce the dangers posed to children on roads.

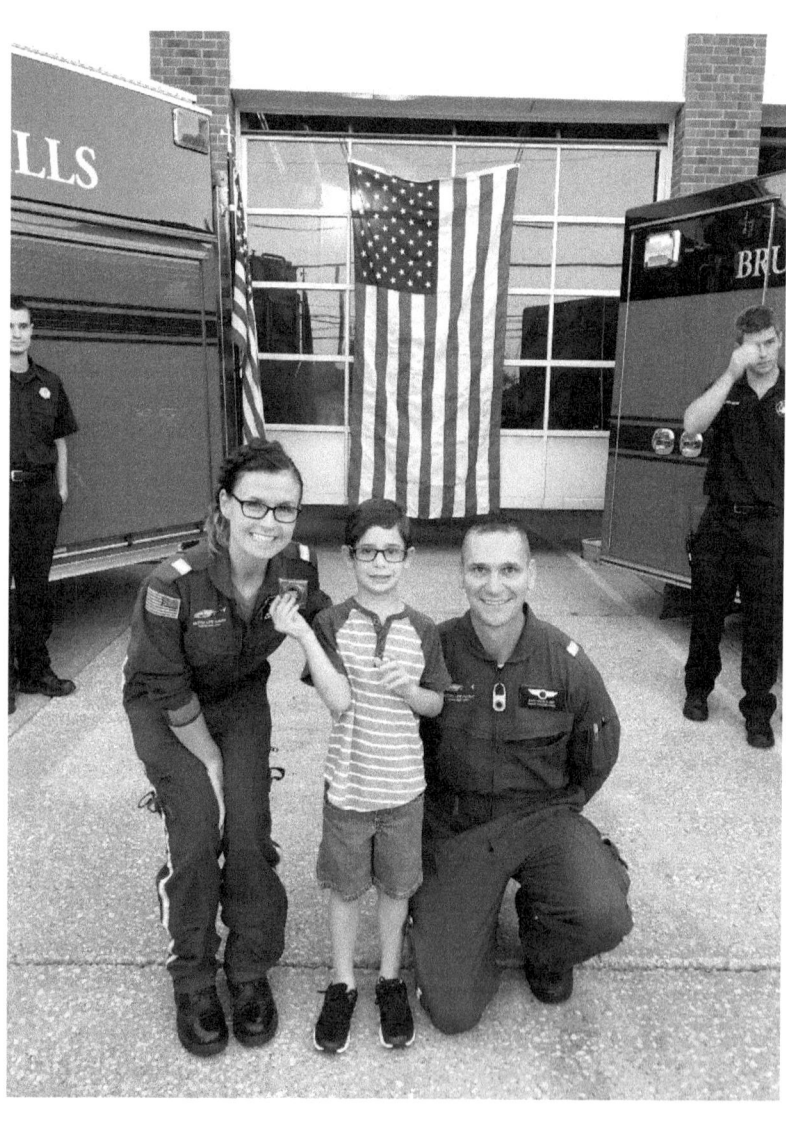

ECHOES OF SILENCE

In a quiet suburban town, there lived a man named Thomas. He was a hardworking father and husband, dedicated to providing for his family and keeping them safe. Thomas owned a handgun which he stored securely in their home, away from the eyes of his curious three-year-old son, Benjamin.

One busy evening, Thomas returned home from shooting at the range, preoccupied with thoughts of an important deadline. Believing he had unloaded the firearm, he absentmindedly placed it on the kitchen table, intending to secure it in its usual location shortly after. However, unbeknownst to him, a single bullet remained in the chamber. As he began preparing dinner, he received an urgent call from his boss. Distracted, he stepped outside to take the call, completely forgetting about the weapon he had left on the table.

Meanwhile, little Benjamin was playing with his toys in the living room when he suddenly noticed the shiny object on the kitchen table. Intrigued, he toddled into the kitchen and climbed onto a chair to get a closer look at the fascinating item.

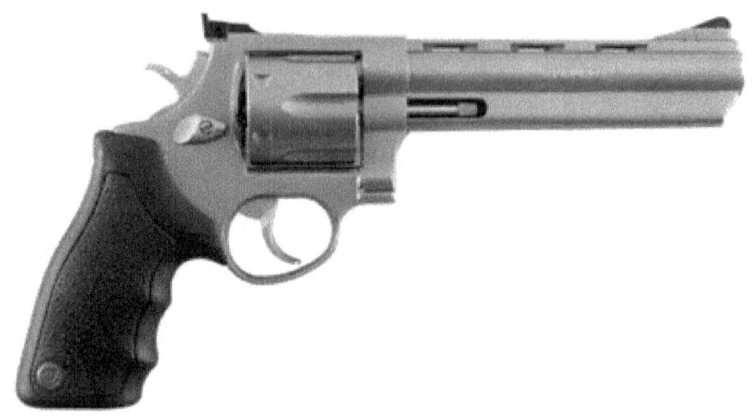

With the cold metal in his small hands, Benjamin began to play with the gun, oblivious to the dangerous power it held. In a split second, his tiny fingers wrapped around the trigger, and a deafening bang reverberated through the house.

Hearing the gunshot, Thomas's heart stopped in terror. Dropping the phone, he raced back inside, desperately calling out for his son. When he reached the kitchen, he found Benjamin lying motionless on the floor, blood surrounding his head, and he immediately called 911.

The local Emergency Medical Services (EMS) team received a frantic call from a distraught father named Thomas, reporting that his three-year-old son, Benjamin, had accidentally shot himself in the head with a loaded gun. Time was of the essence, and both the EMS and Life Flight teams were immediately dispatched to the scene.

The EMS team, with sirens blaring and lights flashing, raced through the streets, navigating the quickest route to reach Benjamin. Meanwhile, the Life Flight team prepared for takeoff, knowing that every second counted in such critical situations. As they took to the skies, the highly skilled crew hoped against all odds that they would arrive in time to save the young boy's life.

Back at the scene, Thomas held his lifeless son in his arms, praying for a miracle as he anxiously awaited the emergency responders. The pain and guilt weighed heavily on him, knowing that his momentary carelessness had led to this horrific event.

When the EMS team arrived, they quickly assessed the situation and began administering life-saving measures to Benjamin. They carefully stabilized his neck, applied pressure to the wound, and administered oxygen. His tiny body was fragile and still, but they clung to the hope that they could save him.

Moments later, the Life Flight helicopter descended from the sky, landing gracefully on a nearby field. The flight team rushed to the scene, their faces etched with determination. They swiftly transferred Benjamin onto a stretcher, securing him for the flight to the nearest Trauma Center.

Before leaving for the hospital, the Life Flight team had to intubate Benjamin to ensure he could breathe properly. They explained the procedure to his father in simple terms: "We need to place a tube down his throat to help him breathe. This will keep his airway open and allow us to give him the oxygen he needs." They carefully inserted the tube, making sure it was secure and functioning correctly.

As the helicopter soared through the air, the medical team worked tirelessly to keep Benjamin alive. They monitored his vital signs, administered fluids, and prepared for any complications that might arise. The minutes turned into an agonizing eternity as they battled against time and the severity of Benjamin's injuries.

Upon arrival at the hospital, Benjamin was immediately taken into the operating room. A team of skilled surgeons and nurses worked diligently to repair the damage caused by the bullet. They fought to control the bleeding, relieve the pressure on his brain, and restore his vital functions.

For hours, the medical team worked tirelessly, their every move guided by a desperate hope. Thomas and his wife waited anxiously in the waiting room, their hearts heavy with fear and guilt. They prayed for a miracle, clinging to the belief that their little boy would pull through.

Despite the medical team's best efforts, Benjamin's condition continued to deteriorate. The damage to his brain was too severe, and his little body was unable to withstand the trauma. As the surgeons worked to repair the damage, Benjamin's heart rate began to slow, and his blood pressure dropped.

The lead surgeon, a seasoned professional with years of experience, made the difficult decision to stop the operation. He knew that continuing would be futile and would only prolong Benjamin's suffering. With a heavy heart, he informed the rest of the team that they had done everything they could.

Benjamin's parents were called into the operating room to say their final goodbyes. They held their son's hand, tears streaming down their faces, as they whispered words of love and comfort. Benjamin passed away peacefully, surrounded by his loving parents and the dedicated medical team who had fought so hard to save him. The loss of their son was a devastating blow to Thomas and his wife, and they would never fully recover from the pain of that day.

The importance of children and gun safety cannot be overstated, as it is a critical aspect of protecting the lives and well-being of our youngest and most vulnerable members of society. Firearms, when not handled or stored properly, can lead to devastating accidents and tragedies involving children. By implementing and promoting gun safety measures, we can significantly reduce the risk of such incidents and build a safer environment for children.

Education: Educating both children and adults about gun safety is essential in preventing accidents. Children should be taught from a young age to respect firearms, understand the potential dangers they pose, and know what to do if they encounter a gun (e.g., not touching it and informing an adult). Adults should also be educated on proper gun handling, storage, and safety measures to ensure that they are responsible gun owners.

Safe storage: One of the most effective ways to prevent accidents involving children and firearms is by securely storing guns and ammunition. Guns should be kept unloaded and locked in a gun safe, cabinet, or other secure storage devices, with the ammunition stored separately. This ensures that children cannot accidentally access or discharge a firearm.

Supervision and guidance: Parents and guardians play a crucial role in ensuring their children's safety around firearms. It is important for them to supervise their children closely and provide clear guidance on the appropriate behavior around guns. If a family owns firearms or participates in activities involving guns, parents should take the time to explain the rules and responsibilities associated with firearms and ensure their children understand the importance of gun safety.

Community involvement: Promoting gun safety within the community can help raise awareness and create a safer environment for children. This can involve supporting local initiatives, such as gun safety courses, public awareness campaigns, and school programs that educate children about the dangers of firearms and the importance of responsible gun ownership.

By prioritizing children's safety and taking the necessary precautions, we can help prevent tragic accidents involving guns and create a safer environment for our children to grow and thrive. The responsibility falls on parents, educators, and the community as a whole to ensure that gun safety is taken seriously and that appropriate measures are put in place to protect our youngest citizens.

RACE AGAINST FATE

Jerry, a 17-year-old car enthusiast, had always been fascinated by automobiles. His passion for cars started at a young age, fueled by countless hours spent watching his father work on their family car. He eagerly absorbed every bit of knowledge his father shared, from the intricacies of engine mechanics to the artistry of bodywork.

Jerry's passion soon evolved into a hands-on hobby. He spent countless hours tinkering with engines, making modifications, and watching YouTube tutorials to learn more about his beloved craft. His bedroom was filled with car magazines, tools, and spare parts, a testament to his dedication.

This particular Saturday was no different, as he eagerly began working on his latest project - an old, rusty car he had picked up at a bargain price. The car, a classic Ford Mustang, had seen better days, but Jerry saw its potential. He had spent weeks meticulously planning its restoration, researching the necessary parts, and gathering the required tools.

Jerry took great care in organizing his workspace before starting the project, ensuring that everything was conveniently within reach. He laid out his tools, arranged the spare parts, and double-checked his reference materials. He was determined to do everything right, to bring the Mustang back to its former glory.

The car was hoisted on jacks, and Jerry slid under it to start working on the engine. He was so engrossed in his task, his mind buzzing with ideas and plans, that he barely noticed the subtle creaking sounds coming from the jacks. Before he knew it, the car gave way, falling on top of him and pinning him underneath its immense weight.

Jerry's mother, who was inside the house, heard the loud crash and rushed out to the garage. She gasped in horror when she saw her son trapped under the car, struggling to breathe. Panicking, she immediately called Emergency Medical Services (EMS) for help.

Within minutes, EMS arrived at the scene and worked swiftly to free Jerry from under the car. They assessed his condition and decided that he needed to be transported to a hospital immediately. As they loaded him into the ambulance, they realized that Jerry's injuries were severe and required specialized care at a Trauma Center.

The decision was made to call for a Life Flight, as it was the fastest way to transport Jerry to the Trauma Center. As the helicopter approached, the EMS team prepared Jerry for the flight.

With precision, the flight crew fastened Jerry to a state-of-the-art stretcher. They took utmost care to stabilize his neck and spine, using a cervical collar and immobilization techniques to prevent further injury. Simultaneously, they connected him to an array of cutting-edge monitors that would help them keep a close watch on his vital signs throughout the flight.

The Life Flight helicopter took off, and the medical team on board worked tirelessly to stabilize Jerry. The cabin was filled with a symphony of beeps and hums from the medical equipment, creating an atmosphere of both urgency and control.

The flight nurse, with years of experience in high-stress situations, vigilantly kept an eye on Jerry's oxygen levels, blood pressure, and heart rate. She adjusted the flow of oxygen through the mask covering his face, ensuring it would compensate for the lower oxygen levels at altitude.

Meanwhile, the paramedic - a veteran of countless rescue missions - administered pain relief and essential fluids through an IV line. His steady hands moved with the precision of a surgeon, despite the helicopter's vibrations and occasional turbulence.

As they monitored Jerry's condition, the medical team exchanged reassuring glances, communicating wordlessly that they had everything under control. They were acutely aware that every passing second was crucial to getting Jerry to the Trauma Center, and they couldn't afford even the slightest delay.

Outside the helicopter, the world seemed to race by in a blur of landscapes as the pilot expertly navigated through the skies. Despite the seriousness of the situation, the beauty of the setting sun cast a warm glow inside the cabin, offering a brief moment of tranquility amidst the chaos.

With each passing mile, the medical team's dedication and expertise were giving Jerry the best possible chance at recovery. And as the Trauma Center's helipad came into view, hope began to rise like the sun on a new day.

As the Life Flight helicopter approached the Trauma Center, the hospital's emergency team was already in position, awaiting Jerry's arrival. The medical staff had been briefed on his condition, and they were prepared for a seamless handoff from the helicopter crew.

The helicopter touched down on the helipad with a gust of wind, signaling the beginning of the next chapter in Jerry's journey to recovery. The flight nurse and paramedic carefully wheeled Jerry out of the helicopter and onto the rooftop, where the hospital's emergency team met them.

Dr. Thompson, a renowned trauma surgeon with a warm smile that put patients at ease, took charge of Jerry's care. She quickly assessed his condition and conferred with the flight nurse before leading the team into the hospital. As they rushed through the corridors, Dr. Thompson barked out orders with an air of authority, ensuring that each member of her team knew their role in Jerry's treatment plan.

Upon reaching the operating room, the team worked with swift precision, transferring Jerry onto the surgical table, and connecting him to the necessary equipment. Dr. Thompson scrubbed in, her years of experience evident in the confidence with which she approached the surgery.

As Dr. Thompson began the delicate procedure, she was acutely aware of the weight of responsibility on her shoulders. Jerry's life was in her hands, and she was committed to doing everything she could to rescue him. With every incision and suture, she fought against time, knowing that every minute mattered.

Hours passed, and the tense atmosphere in the operating room gradually gave way to cautious optimism. Dr. Thompson and her team had successfully addressed Jerry's most critical injuries, and now it was a matter of monitoring his progress and ensuring his body could heal itself.

Jerry was moved to the intensive care unit, where he remained under close observation for several days. His mother sat by his side, offering unwavering support and love. Slowly but surely, Jerry began to regain consciousness, his body responding positively to the expert care he had received.

Over the following weeks, Jerry continued to improve, astounding the medical staff with his determination and resilience. His mother's constant presence provided him with the emotional support he needed to push through the pain and setbacks.

As Jerry grew stronger, he was moved to a regular hospital room, where he began an intensive rehabilitation program. The physical therapists marveled at his progress, witnessing firsthand his passion for life and his eagerness to get back to his beloved cars.

Finally, the day came when Dr. Thompson, beaming with pride, announced that Jerry was ready to go home. With tears in her eyes, she embraced Jerry and his mother, congratulating them on the incredible journey they had just completed.

Jerry's recovery was nothing short of miraculous. As he left the hospital, he knew that he owed his life to the remarkable team of medical professionals who had worked tirelessly to save him. And although his road to full recovery would be long and challenging, Jerry was filled with gratitude and hope for the future, eager to return to his passion for cars and embrace the adventures that awaited him.

Working on an automobile can be a rewarding experience, but it's crucial to prioritize safety during maintenance or repairs. A common mistake is relying solely on jacks or using underrated jacks to support the vehicle without proper securing. This can pose serious dangers. Always use jack stands in addition to jacks and ensure the vehicle is on a flat, stable surface to prevent accidents.

Vehicle instability: Jacks are primarily designed for lifting and lowering a vehicle, not for long-term support. When a car is supported only by jacks, it may become unstable, making it prone to tipping or falling.

Jack failure: Jacks, like any other mechanical device, can fail due to wear, manufacturing defects, or improper use. If a jack fails while you're working underneath the vehicle, it can cause severe injuries or even be fatal.

Uneven weight distribution: When using jacks alone, the weight of the vehicle may not be evenly distributed, causing excessive pressure on certain points. This can lead to the vehicle slipping or falling off the jacks unexpectedly.

Limited access: Relying on jacks alone restricts your ability to move around and access all areas of the vehicle comfortably. This can lead to awkward positioning and increased chances of accidents.

Improper lifting: If the vehicle is not lifted correctly, it can damage the vehicle's frame, suspension components, or other parts. Additionally, improper lifting can contribute to the vehicle becoming unstable on the jacks.

To mitigate these risks, it's essential to follow proper safety procedures:

Use jack stands: After lifting the vehicle with a jack, always use sturdy, well-rated jack stands to support its weight. Place them under the designated lift points on the vehicle's frame for maximum stability.

Chock the wheels: Prevent the vehicle from rolling by placing wheel chocks behind the tires that remain on the ground.

Work on a flat, solid surface: Ensure that the area where you're working is level and made of solid material, such as concrete. This helps prevent the jacks or jack stands from sinking or shifting.

Inspect your equipment: Regularly check your jacks and jack stands for signs of wear, damage, or corrosion. Replace any equipment that appears compromised.

Lower the vehicle carefully: When you're finished with your repairs, lower the vehicle slowly and cautiously to avoid sudden movements or shifts in weight.

By following these safety measures and using the proper equipment, you can significantly reduce the dangers associated with working on an automobile.

THE UNSEEN DOSE

In a small, quaint town, there lived a curious young girl named Olivia. She had a loving family, and she was particularly close to her grandmother, who lived with them. Her grandmother had been suffering from high blood pressure for quite some time now and took medication to manage her condition.

One sunny afternoon, Olivia's parents were away at work, and she was spending time with her grandmother. As her grandmother took her daily blood pressure pills, Olivia couldn't help but wonder what would happen if she took one of these magical pills herself. In her mind, they seemed like tiny superheroes, protecting her grandmother from harm.

As soon as her grandmother left the room, Olivia seized the opportunity to investigate the pills. One by one, she shook them out of the bottle and examined them closely. They looked so harmless, like little candies. Before she knew it, she had impulsively swallowed one down.

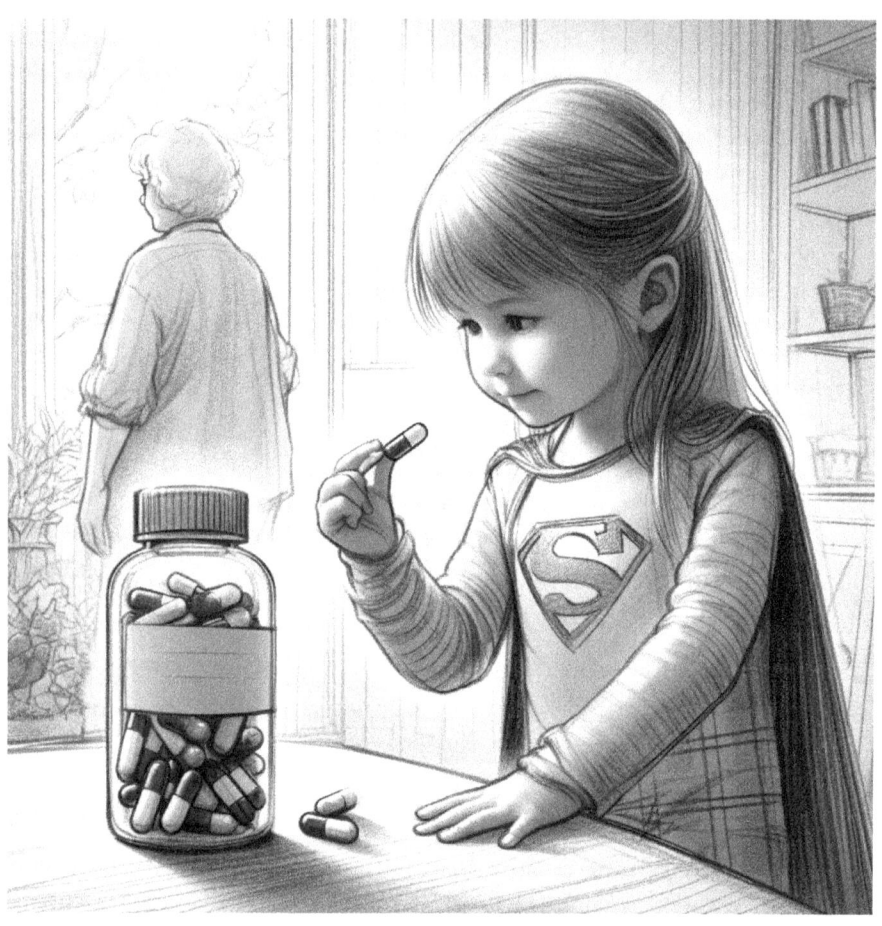

Unknown to Olivia and her grandmother, the effects of the pill began to take hold gradually. About thirty minutes after swallowing the pill, Olivia started to feel a bit off. At first, it was just a slight dizziness, something she thought might pass. She continued playing, but the feeling persisted and slowly intensified.

After about forty-five minutes, Olivia's dizziness grew worse, and she began to feel lightheaded. Her vision started to blur, making it difficult for her to focus on anything. She tried to shake it off, but the symptoms only worsened.

In just an hour, Olivia's condition declined drastically. Her grandmother found the open bottle of pills and wondered if Olivia had consumed any of them.

Olivia felt an overwhelming sense of weakness, her heart slower than usual. Panic set in as she realized something was seriously wrong. She stumbled into the living room, her movements unsteady, and her breathing labored.

Her grandmother, noticing Olivia's distress, rushed to her side. Seeing her granddaughter's pale face and unfocused eyes, she immediately knew something was terribly wrong. With trembling hands, she called 911, her voice filled with fear and urgency as she explained the situation to the operator.

The Emergency Medical Services (EMS) arrived quickly, assessing Olivia's condition and rushing her to the nearest small hospital. As they wheeled her into the emergency room, Olivia's heart suddenly stopped. The medical staff sprang into action, performing CPR on her fragile body. Every second felt like an eternity. After a lengthy period of performing CPR, the medical teams were able to regain a pulse.

Despite their best efforts, the hospital staff realized that Olivia needed specialized care. They made the decision to call for a Life Flight to transport her to a larger hospital with advanced facilities. As the helicopter approached, the whirring of its blades filled the air, drowning out everything else.

Olivia's grandmother had arrived by this time and clutched her hand tightly, whispering words of love and encouragement. Tears streamed down her face as she prayed with all her heart that her precious granddaughter would pull through this terrifying ordeal. Her voice trembled with emotion, each word a plea for Olivia's recovery.

As the Life Flight team carefully loaded Olivia onto the helicopter, her grandmother took one last look at her brave little girl. She whispered, "Stay strong, my love," her voice breaking with the weight of her emotions.

With that, the helicopter lifted off, carrying Olivia towards the life-saving care she so desperately needed. The townspeople looked on, their hearts heavy with concern but filled with hope for Olivia's recovery.

As the Life Flight disappeared into the horizon, the sun began to set, casting a warm, golden glow over the town. It was as if nature itself was offering a promise: that no matter how challenging the times, there would always be a new dawn waiting to bring light and hope once again.

As the helicopter soared through the sky, the Life Flight team, consisting of a skilled paramedic and a dedicated nurse, worked tirelessly to stabilize Olivia's condition. The duo monitored her vital signs, ensuring that she received the necessary oxygen and medications.

In the tight cabin, the paramedic and nurse exchanged glances, silently communicating while working to save Olivia. They had seen countless patients in critical conditions before, but something about this young girl's spirit touched them deeply. It was as if her strength and determination radiated from her fragile body, willing her to survive.

Olivia's mind drifted in and out of consciousness, her thoughts a blur of memories and dreams. She could feel the steady vibrations of the helicopter beneath her, and the gentle touch of the paramedic and nurse working to keep her alive. Somewhere deep inside, she knew that her grandmother's love was with her, providing her with the strength to fight for her life.

As the helicopter neared its destination, the cityscape came into view, guiding the way to salvation. The pilot expertly maneuvered the aircraft, touching down on the helipad atop the larger hospital.

The Life Flight team carefully transferred Olivia onto a gurney and swiftly moved her into the hospital. Inside, the doctors took over, their eyes filled with hope and determination. The paramedic and nurse shared a solemn nod with the doctors, knowing that Olivia's journey was far from over, but they had done everything in their power to give her a fighting chance.

As the helicopter lifted off once more, returning to the skies, the paramedic and nurse couldn't help but think of Olivia and her brave spirit. They knew that her story would stay with them forever, a reminder of the preciousness of life and the power of hope. Departing into the sky, they quietly wished her the best, recognizing the deep impression she had left on them.

Olivia was immediately taken to a specialized pediatric intensive care unit, where a team of highly skilled doctors and nurses were waiting to attend to her. They quickly assessed her condition and determined the best course of action to reverse the effects of the blood pressure pills she had ingested.

Working together, they administered the appropriate treatments to counteract the drug's impact on Olivia's body. Hours passed as they monitored her progress closely, observing every change in her vital signs and adjusting their approach accordingly. Olivia's grandmother replayed every moment of the day, wondering how she hadn't noticed Olivia's interest in the pills. The thought of losing her granddaughter over something so preventable was almost too much to bear.

Gradually, Olivia's heart rate stabilized, and her blood pressure returned to normal levels. The color returned to her cheeks, and her breathing grew steady and even. The medical team was amazed by her incredible recovery, as it was rare for patients in such critical conditions to bounce back so quickly.

As the days went by, Olivia continued to regain her strength. Her family, especially her grandmother, stayed by her side throughout this challenging time, offering love, support, and encouragement. The hospital staff marveled at the young girl's resilience and determination, attributing her remarkable recovery to her unwavering spirit.

Soon, Olivia was well enough to be discharged from the hospital. As she left the building, she was greeted by the warm sunlight which seemed to celebrate her victory over adversity. Her family and the medical team exchanged heartfelt goodbyes, knowing that they had witnessed a true miracle.

The safety and well-being of our children are of paramount importance, and one crucial aspect of ensuring their protection is preventing their unsupervised access to medications. With the ever-increasing prevalence of prescription and over-the-counter drugs in modern households, it is essential to be vigilant about medication storage, usage, and disposal. Unintentional ingestion of these substances can lead to severe health consequences, including life-threatening emergencies and long-term complications. By proactively implementing strategies to keep medications out of children's reach and educating them about the potential dangers, we can significantly reduce the risk of accidental poisonings and foster a secure environment for our young ones to grow and thrive.

Store medications securely: Keep all medications, including over-the-counter drugs, vitamins, and supplements, in a locked cabinet or out of reach of children. Child-resistant containers are not foolproof, so it's essential to store them safely.

Keep medications in their original containers: This helps avoid confusion between different types of medications and allows you to quickly identify the contents in case of an emergency.

Educate children about medication safety: Teach children that medications are not candy and should only be taken when given by an adult. Explain the importance of taking medicine as prescribed and the potential dangers of ingesting unknown substances.

Be vigilant during travel or visits: When staying at someone else's home or traveling, ensure that medications are stored securely and out of sight. Don't leave medications in purses, bags, or on countertops where children can easily access them.

Dispose of expired or unused medications properly: Follow local guidelines for disposing of medications, such as taking them to a pharmacy or designated drop-off location. Do not flush medications down the toilet or throw them in the trash, as this can lead to contamination of water supplies and harm wildlife.

Be prepared for emergencies: Keep the Poison Control Center's phone number (1-800-222-1222 in the United States) saved in your phone and posted in a visible location in your home. In case of accidental ingestion, call for help immediately.

Monitor medication usage: Keep track of how much medication is in each container to detect if any has gone missing or been tampered with.

Set a good example: Always take your own medications responsibly and demonstrate proper medication storage and disposal habits.

Remember, prevention is the key to ensuring medication safety around children. By following these guidelines, you can help reduce the risk of accidental ingestion and create a safer environment for everyone.

A MOMENT OF FRUSTRATION

William was over the moon when his son was born. He had always wanted a child, and now that he was holding his new baby boy in his arms, he felt like everything was right in the world. He spent every moment he could with his son, playing with him, changing his diapers, and watching him grow.

But as time went on, William found himself becoming increasingly frustrated with his young son. The sleepless nights and constant crying were taking a toll on him, and he found himself snapping at the little boy more often than he'd like to admit.

One evening, after a particularly long day at work, William was trying to soothe his son who had been crying for hours. No matter what he did, the baby just wouldn't stop crying. In a moment of frustration, William shook his son.

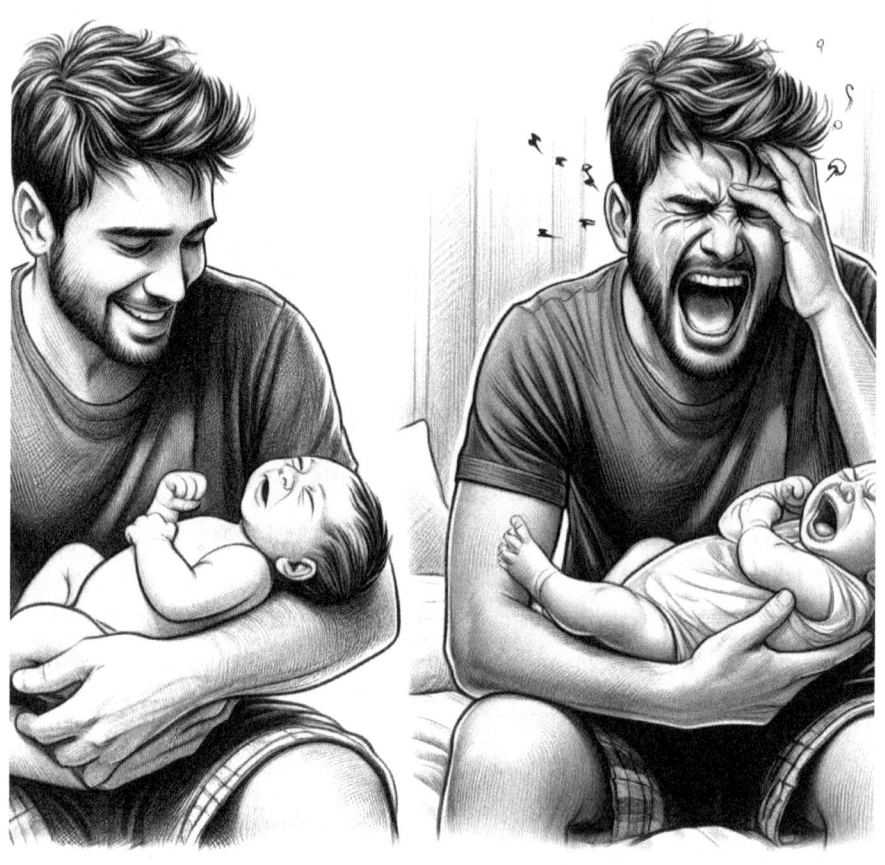

But as soon as he did it, he knew he had made a mistake. He could feel the tiny body in his hands going limp, and he quickly put his son down and called for an ambulance.

The ambulance arrived in minutes, and the paramedics immediately assessed the condition of William's son. They quickly realized that the baby's condition was critical. He needed to be transported to a hospital with advanced pediatric care, so they called for a Life Flight helicopter to transport the infant.

As they waited for the Life Flight helicopter to arrive, the paramedics worked quickly to stabilize the infant's condition. They carefully monitored his breathing and heart rate, adjusting his treatment as necessary to keep him alive. William observed anxiously as the medical professionals worked to save his son's life, experiencing a sense of helplessness and terror.

The paramedics communicated with the Life Flight crew, giving them updates on the infant's condition and preparing them for what to expect when they arrived. They knew that time was of the essence, and they did everything in their power to ensure that the baby received the best possible care while waiting for transport.

Upon the arrival of the Life Flight helicopter, Sarah and Tom, a flight nurse and flight paramedic respectively, took charge of the infant's care. Both Sarah and Tom were fully aware of the seriousness of the situation and promptly fitted their monitoring equipment before transferring the baby onto the helicopter.

As the helicopter lifted off the ground, Sarah and Tom recognized the importance of every passing moment. The young child was in critical condition. His tiny body lay limp on the stretcher in the back of the helicopter, with machines beeping rhythmically around him.

Sarah took charge of the child's care, while Tom prepared the necessary medications and equipment. As they flew over the countryside, Sarah monitored the child's breathing closely. The child's breathing became increasingly labored, and Sarah knew that she needed to act fast.

Sarah acted quickly and grabbed the required equipment, placing a breathing tube to assist with his respiration. She worked quickly and efficiently, her movements precise and focused. Tom supported her by providing her with medical instruments and closely monitoring the child's vital signs.

The Life Flight transport was already chaotic, but now the urgency had significantly increased. The sound of the helicopter blades seemed louder as they tried to keep the child stable. Sarah and Tom both worked together seamlessly, knowing that the child's life was in their hands.

Sarah used the radio to inform the hospital staff that they were on their way with a critically ill patient who had a breathing tube. Upon their arrival, she specifically requested that a ventilator be ready and present in the room. The helicopter touched down smoothly, and the team rushed the child into the emergency room.

The next few days were a blur for William. His son was in critical condition, and he spent every moment he could by his side, praying that he would pull through. The guilt and shame he felt were overwhelming, and he couldn't believe he had hurt the one person he loved more than anything in the world.

Thankfully, William's son did eventually recover from his injuries. But the incident changed William forever. He knew he could never let his frustration get the best of him again, and he worked hard to control his temper and be a better father to his son.

The incident also had serious legal ramifications for William. He was investigated by child protective services and faced potential charges of child abuse. William cooperated fully with the investigation, admitting his mistake, and expressing deep remorse for his actions. He was placed on probation for two years and required to attend parenting classes and undergo counseling as part of his probation. His probation officer, Mr. Davis, became a regular presence in William's life, conducting home visits and monitoring his progress.

During his probation, William faced many challenges. He struggled with feelings of guilt and shame, often replaying the incident in his mind and wondering how he could have let his emotions get the better of him. Despite these challenges, William's love for his son became the driving force behind his efforts to change. He attended every parenting class with dedication, eager to learn how to be the best father he could be.

William's son was the most important part of his life. Every day, he made a conscious effort to show his son how much he loved him. He spent quality time with him, playing games and simply being present.

William's journey was not easy, but his unwavering love for his son gave him the strength to overcome his past mistakes. He knew that his son's well-being and happiness were worth every effort and sacrifice. Through his actions, William demonstrated that his son was, and always would be, the most important part of his life.

Shaken baby syndrome (SBS) is a serious and life-threatening condition that can occur if an infant or young child is shaken violently. The shaking can cause bleeding in the brain and lead to permanent brain damage, blindness, seizures, or even death.

One of the primary causes of SBS is the caregiver losing their temper and becoming frustrated with the infant's crying or fussiness. It's important to remember that infants cry as a means of communication, and it's not a behavior that can be controlled or stopped by the caregiver.

The risks of losing your temper and shaking a baby are significant and can include severe consequences for both the baby and the caregiver. In addition to the physical and emotional trauma that can result from SBS, the caregiver may also face legal charges and social stigma.

To prevent SBS, it's essential to understand the dangers of shaking a baby and to take steps to manage your emotions and frustrations. Here are some tips to help prevent SBS:

Take breaks: Caregiving can be stressful and overwhelming, so it's essential to take breaks when needed. If you feel yourself becoming frustrated or overwhelmed, step away from the baby and take a few deep breaths or engage in a relaxing activity.

Don't work all night and plan to watch the children when you're tired: Try to ensure you are well-rested before caring for your child. Working long hours or pulling all-nighters and then watching your children the next day can lead to fatigue and increase the risk of losing your temper or making poor decisions.

Seek support: Don't be afraid to ask for help or seek support from family members, friends, or healthcare professionals. Caring for an infant can be challenging, and it's okay to ask for assistance.

Learn coping strategies: Try to develop healthy coping strategies for stress, such as exercise, meditation, or talking to a trusted friend or counselor.

Understand infant development: Learn about infant development and understand that crying is a normal part of a baby's communication. It's not a deliberate attempt to frustrate or upset the caregiver.

By taking these steps, caregivers can prevent SBS and provide a safe and nurturing environment for infants and young children.

WATCH YOUR BACK

On a scorching summer day in a peaceful suburban neighborhood, the air was filled with the sounds of children's laughter and the distant hum of lawnmowers. Grandpa, a retired mechanic with a love for gardening, was meticulously mowing his expansive lawn, the sweat glistening on his brow under the blazing sun. Nearby, Grandma, a retired schoolteacher with a warm smile and a twinkle in her eye, was hosting a delightful tea party for their three-year-old granddaughter, Autumn.

Autumn, a bright and curious child with boundless energy, was captivated by the miniature tea set and the assortment of stuffed animals gathered around her on the patio table. She giggled as Grandma poured imaginary tea into tiny porcelain cups and pretended to sip from her own, her pinky finger raised delicately in the air. The two of them were lost in their own little world, oblivious to the potential danger lurking nearby.

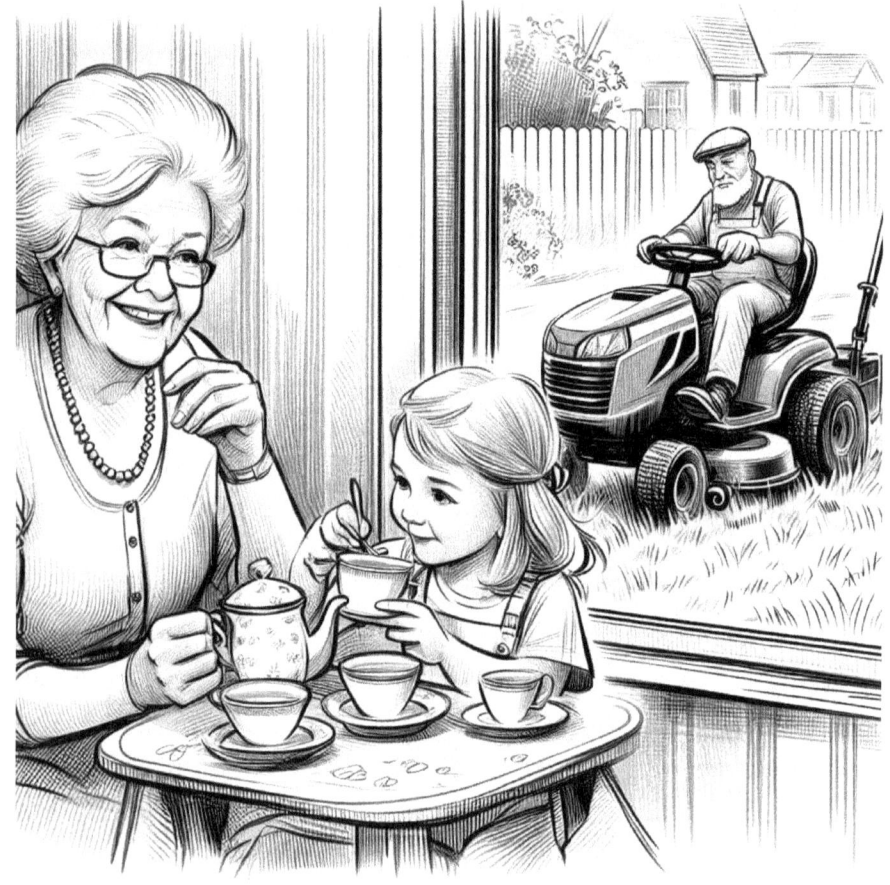

Suddenly, Grandma remembered that she had left a batch of cookies in the oven. Excusing herself with a quick kiss on Autumn's forehead, she hurried inside, leaving the little girl momentarily unattended. Autumn, her attention span fleeting, quickly grew bored with the tea party. The rhythmic whirring of the lawnmower in the distance caught her attention, and she decided to investigate.

Unbeknownst to Autumn, Grandpa had just finished mowing the main lawn and was now maneuvering his riding mower around a flower bed, carefully trimming the edges. He was so focused on his task that he didn't hear Autumn's approaching footsteps or her excited squeals as she ran towards him.

In a split second, tragedy struck. A horrifying thud and a chilling silence filled the air as Grandpa turned to discover his beloved granddaughter lying motionless on the ground, the victim of a terrible accident. The vibrant colors of the flower bed seemed to fade as a wave of nausea washed over him.

At first, Grandpa didn't even realize what had happened; he quickly turned off the lawnmower and ran to Autumn's side. She was crying and in a lot of pain. Grandpa was devastated. He had never felt so helpless in his life.

Wasting no time, Grandpa called 911. The ambulance arrived within minutes, and upon assessing the injuries, knew the situation called for immediate action. Without hesitation, the EMTs called for a medical helicopter.

By the time the flight crew arrived, the ambulance crew had already loaded Autumn onto a stretcher and into the ambulance. She was in severe pain, her small body wracked with sobs as her grandparents stood by, their faces etched with worry and fear. The flight nurse and paramedic quickly assessed the situation, their trained eyes taking in the extent of Autumn's injuries.

The flight nurse, a compassionate and experienced professional, knelt beside Autumn, speaking to her in a soft, reassuring voice. He explained that they were going to take her on a helicopter ride to a special hospital where doctors would help her feel better. Autumn, though frightened, seemed to understand and nodded bravely as the paramedic gently placed a stuffed animal in her arms.

While the helicopter took off, Autumn's grandparents watched in horror, their hearts filled with a mix of hope and dread. They could only pray that their precious granddaughter would pull through.

Inside the helicopter, the medical team worked tirelessly to keep Autumn stable and alive. The flight nurse administered pain medication and fluids through an IV, while the paramedic monitored her vital signs, watching for any changes that might indicate a worsening condition.

The flight was a blur of noise and activity, but the medical team remained calm and focused, their movements precise and efficient. They knew that every second counted and that their young patient's life depended on their expertise.

As the helicopter approached the hospital, the flight nurse radioed ahead, providing the medical team on the ground with an update on Autumn's condition. The landing was smooth, and the medical team wasted no time in transferring Autumn to a waiting ambulance for the short ride to the emergency room.

Grandpa was overcome by the immense weight of guilt and shame. He couldn't believe that he had been so careless; neglecting to check if Autumn was nearby. He knew he would never forgive himself for what had happened, no matter the outcome.

Days passed slowly as Grandpa waited for news about Autumn's condition. He couldn't eat or sleep, and the image of her injured on the ground haunted him day and night. When he finally received the news that she was on the road to recovery, he was overcome with emotion. A weight was lifted from his shoulders, but the scars of the accident remained.

From that day on, Grandpa was a changed man. He became more withdrawn, no longer the jovial and carefree person he once was. He would often sit alone in his backyard, staring at the spot where the accident had occurred. His wife tried to console him, but nothing seemed to help. The guilt and shame consumed him, and he felt like he didn't deserve to be happy again.

Whenever Grandpa mowed the lawn, the sound of the blades became a haunting reminder of the tragic event. The image of Autumn's little shoes abandoned in the grass, the agony on her face, and the dreadful understanding that he was to blame would be etched in his mind. Each night, he lay awake, staring at the ceiling, wondering if there was a way he could ever forgive himself.

It wasn't until one day when Autumn came to visit him at home that something shifted. She ran towards him, calling out "Grandpa!" with joy in her voice. She hugged him tightly, and Grandpa realized that he still had a chance to make things right. He made it his mission to spend as much time with her as possible, cherishing every moment they had together.

Over time, the scars began to heal. Grandpa learned to forgive himself and to find joy in life once again. He still thought about the accident, but it no longer defined him. Instead, he viewed it as a way to consistently remind himself to be cautious in the presence of young children and to value the time spent with his loved ones.

In the end, the accident brought Grandpa and Autumn even closer together. It was a painful lesson to learn, but it reminded him of the importance of family and the preciousness of life.

Checking behind a lawnmower or automobile before backing up with small children is extremely important and cannot be underestimated. This is particularly true for models lacking a rear camera. Lawnmowers and cars can cause serious injuries or even fatalities if proper precautions are not taken.

Small children are especially vulnerable to lawnmower and car accidents because they may not fully understand the dangers posed by the equipment and vehicles. They could run up to the lawnmower or car without realizing the danger and get caught in the blades or struck by the mower deck or vehicle.

For this reason, it's imperative to make it a habit to check behind your lawnmower and automobile before backing up. It only takes a few seconds to do so but doing it every time you need to back up can prevent devastating accidents.

Similar to cars, lawnmower models now come equipped with backup cameras or sensors to assist operators in being more aware of their surroundings. However, it is important to keep in mind that technology can malfunction.

It's also crucial to educate children about the risks associated with lawn equipment, automobiles, and other large equipment, and how to stay safe near them. Children should understand the potential dangers these machines pose, such as severe injuries from lawnmowers or accidents involving cars. Teaching them to maintain a safe distance from these machines, especially when they are in operation, is essential.

Additionally, emphasizing the importance of adult supervision can prevent many accidents. Children should also be instructed on emergency procedures, such as moving away quickly and alerting an adult if something goes wrong.

Encouraging them to be aware of their surroundings and avoid playing in areas where these machines are being used can further enhance their safety. By providing this education, we can help ensure that children understand the potential dangers and know how to stay safe around lawn equipment, automobiles, and other large machinery.

THE MISCALCULATED DIVE

In a small town nestled between green hills and a sparkling lake, lived a vibrant 10-year-old boy named Max. Max was known for his boundless energy and adventurous spirit, always ready to explore every nook and cranny that his little world had to offer.

One scorching summer day, the local community pool beckoned Max and his friends with its promise of cool relief. The pool was alive with laughter and splashing, children of all ages diving, swimming, and playing. Max, with his signature grin, decided to join the fun.

Max was not a proficient swimmer but was always eager to jump into the pool. He loved the feeling of the cool water enveloping him, the momentary silence underneath, and the rush of resurfacing. He would often close his eyes during his dives, savoring the sensation.

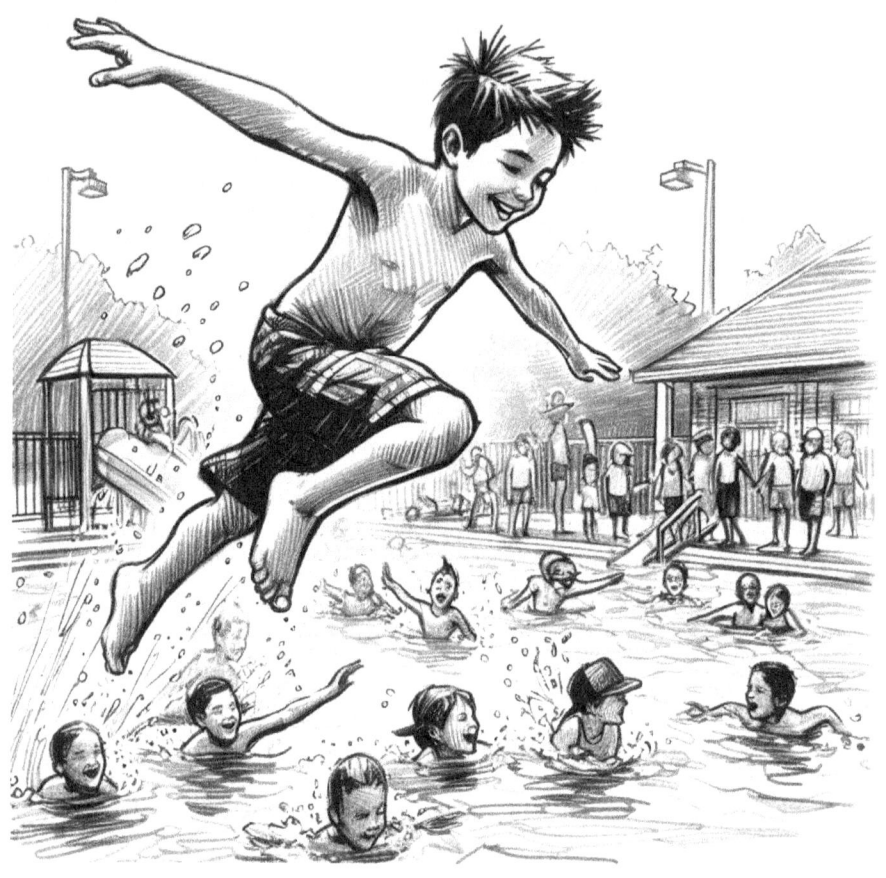

On this fateful day, Max decided to attempt a daring leap. With a running start, he launched himself into the air, aiming for the shallow end of the pool. As he descended, the world seemed to slow down, but an unexpected miscalculation awaited him at the bottom.

Max hit his head hard on the pool's concrete floor. A sharp, searing pain shot through his body, and he found himself unable to move. Panic set in as he struggled to surface, but his body refused to cooperate. The undercurrent of noise and laughter above was quickly replaced by a disconcerting silence and a sense of impending doom.

Above the surface, Max's friends noticed his prolonged absence. One of them spotted his motionless form beneath the water and raised the alarm. The poolside erupted into chaos as lifeguards jumped into action, pulling Max out of the water. His usually flushed face was pale, and his body was limp. The pool, once a source of joy and relief, had turned into a scene of terror.

In the distance, the wailing siren of an ambulance grew louder. The paramedics arrived, their faces grave as they assessed Max's condition. They worked with swift precision, stabilizing his neck and transferring him onto a stretcher. As they loaded him into the ambulance, the crowd watched in stunned silence, their fun-filled day turned into a nightmare.

As the ambulance doors closed, the crowd was left behind, their laughter replaced by prayers for the brave and adventurous Max. His story served as a stark reminder of life's fragility, forever changing the small town's perception of a simple summer's day at the pool.

Inside the ambulance, the atmosphere was charged with a mix of urgency and calm precision. Max lay on the stretcher, his face pale but peaceful, oblivious to the flurry of activity around him. The paramedics worked in tandem, their skilled hands moving effortlessly as they monitored his vitals and kept his neck stable.

The senior paramedic, a weathered man named Frank, knew the magnitude of Max's situation. He made a swift decision, picking up the radio and calling into the hospital. "We've got a critical neck injury," he reported, his voice steady despite the dire situation. "Requesting Life Flight."

The request was granted immediately. A helicopter, specially equipped for medical emergencies, was dispatched from the nearest hospital. Radiating hope, it pierced through the pristine blue sky.

As the ambulance sped towards the designated rendezvous point, Frank explained the situation to Max. Even in his unconscious state, it seemed as though Max could hear Frank's soothing voice, offering reassurance that help was on the way.

The sound of rotors chopping through the air signaled the helicopter. The ambulance screeched to a halt in an open field, and the paramedics swiftly transferred Max onto a stretcher. With utmost care, they carried him towards the waiting helicopter.

The Life Flight team took over, securing Max inside the helicopter. The interior was cramped, filled with medical equipment, but every square inch was designed to preserve life during the crucial golden hour. As the helicopter lifted off, the medical team inside worked tirelessly, keeping a vigilant eye on Max's vitals.

The helicopter cut through the wind, its blades leaving a trail of dust in the open field. Inside, amidst the hum of rotors and the beep of monitors, Max continued to fight. His story was far from over, and his spirit remained unbroken.

The flight was a race against time, the landscape below blurring into an indistinct tapestry of green and blue. As they neared the hospital, the pilot expertly maneuvered the helicopter, landing on the helipad with a gentle thud.

Max's journey was not over yet, but he was one step closer to the help he desperately needed. The helicopter flight, a testament to human ingenuity and compassion, had given him a fighting chance. And, in the face of adversity, that was all Max needed - a chance to fight another day.

The hospital was a flurry of activity as the Life Flight team arrived. A team of doctors and nurses were already waiting, ready to take over. Max was quickly wheeled into the emergency department. The harsh fluorescent lighting and the antiseptic smell were a stark contrast to the sunny poolside where his day had begun. He was surrounded by a team of medical professionals, their faces hidden behind masks, their eyes filled with determination.

Dr. Collins, a well-known neurosurgeon known for his steady hands and unwavering focus, took the lead. He examined Max's scans, his brow furrowed in concentration. It was a complex case, but not hopeless. A glimmer of hope sparked in his eyes - Max had a fighting chance. Dr. Collins quickly outlined a plan to reduce the pressure on Max's spinal cord, knowing that every second counted in preserving Max's mobility.

Hours turned into days as Max underwent multiple surgeries. The hospital became a second home for his family, their days filled with worry but also an unwavering faith in the medical team. Their prayers, along with those of the entire town, echoed through the hospital halls.

Slowly, Max began to show signs of improvement. His vitals stabilized, the swelling in his neck reduced, and one unforgettable afternoon, he moved his fingers. His recovery was nothing short of a miracle, a testament to his resilience and the skill of his doctors.

Max's journey was far from over, but each day brought small victories. From moving his fingers to wiggling his toes, to bending his arms and legs, each achievement was celebrated.

His room was filled with cards and balloons, tangible proof of the love and support that poured in from all corners of the town.

Months later, with the aid of crutches and extensive physical therapy, Max left the hospital, not on a stretcher but on his own two feet. His neck was supported by a brace, a reminder of the ordeal he had been through, but his spirit was undeterred. He was greeted with cheers and tears, a hero in the eyes of his town.

Max's story served as a reminder of the strength of the human spirit and the miracles of modern medicine. His accident at the pool had started a journey filled with fear and uncertainty, but it ended with hope and triumph. The boy who had dived into the shallow end of the pool emerged stronger, forever embodying the spirit of resilience and courage.

Take Home Points

Diving safely in a swimming pool is crucial to prevent injuries. Here are some guidelines to follow:

Check the depth and for obstructions: Always check the depth of the water before diving. It should be deep enough to absorb the diver's momentum. The American Red Cross recommends a minimum of 9 feet. Also, make sure there are no obstructions in the water such as other swimmers, floating toys, or underwater ledges.

Dive in designated areas: Only dive in areas of the pool that are marked for diving. These areas are designed to be deep enough and free from obstructions.

Use proper diving techniques: Enter the water hands first with your arms extended over your head. This helps protect your head and neck.

Never dive alone: Always have someone nearby when you're diving. In case of an accident, they can get help or assist you.

Take diving lessons: If you're new to diving, consider taking lessons from a certified instructor. They can teach you proper techniques and safety measures.

Check the pool's condition: Ensure the pool's water is clear and its bottom is visible. Murky water can hide hazards. Also, check for any signs of damage or wear on the diving board or platform.

Parents play a crucial role in teaching children to dive safely. Here are some tips:

Lead by example: Demonstrate safe diving practices. Children often mimic the behavior of adults, so showing them how to dive safely is essential.

Educate about risks: Explain the potential dangers of diving improperly, such as head and neck injuries. Use age-appropriate language to ensure they understand.

Supervise closely: Always supervise children when they are diving. Be within arm's reach to assist if needed.

Set clear rules: Establish and enforce rules about where and how to dive. Make sure children understand that diving is only allowed in designated areas and never in shallow water.

Encourage practice: Allow children to practice diving in a safe environment under supervision. This helps them build confidence and improve their technique.

Enroll in lessons: Consider enrolling children in diving lessons with a certified instructor. Professional guidance can help them learn proper techniques and safety measures.

Positive reinforcement: Praise children when they follow safety rules and dive correctly. Positive reinforcement encourages them to continue practicing safe behaviors.

By following these guidelines and teaching children about safe diving practices, parents can help prevent injuries and ensure a fun and safe swimming experience.

HEATWAVE HORROR

Once upon a time, in a city full of life and energy, lived a loving father named Jack. Jack was the epitome of a devoted father, his life revolving around his cherubic two-year-old daughter, Sophia. She was his sunshine, her giggles his favorite melody, and her happiness his ultimate goal.

One fateful day, with the sun blazing in the sky, Jack had an unusually hectic schedule at work. He had to prepare for an important presentation, which had been causing him sleepless nights. Despite the stress, he managed to ready Sophia for daycare, packed her favorite lunch, and securely fastened her into the car seat. Sophia, innocent of the world's worries, handed Jack her beloved stuffed bunny, which he absentmindedly placed on the passenger seat next to him.

Lost in thoughts about his presentation, Jack drove the familiar route. However, instead of stopping at the daycare center, he found himself pulling into his office parking lot. He grabbed his briefcase and rushed into the office, forgetting the most precious part of his life inside the hot car.

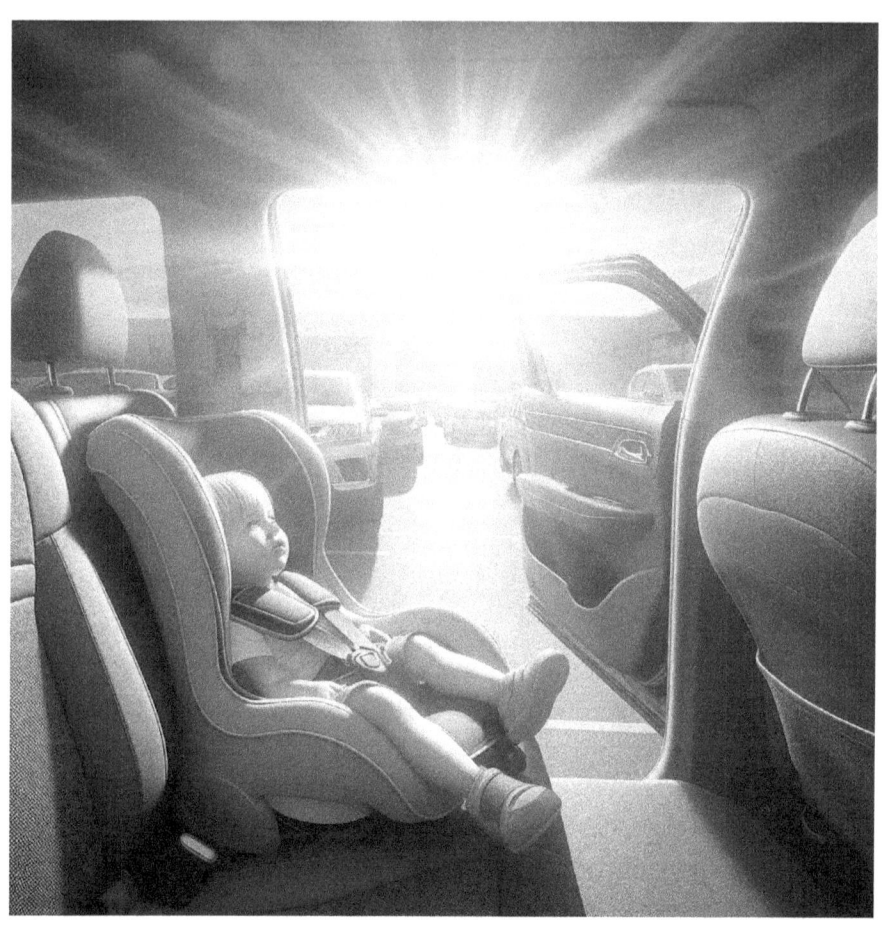

Hours passed as Jack immersed himself in his work, oblivious to the passing time. The moment he saw a photo of Sophia with her stuffed bunny hanging on his wall, he was struck by a sudden realization. His heart pounded in his chest as he sprinted towards the parking lot, praying desperately that Sophia was okay.

He found Sophia unconscious in the back seat, her little body succumbing to the heat. The sight stole his breath away as he dialed 911, tears streaming down his face.

The wail of emergency sirens soon filled the air as paramedics rushed towards Jack's car. They quickly assessed Sophia's condition, their faces grim and focused. Despite their swift and professional attempts to stabilize her, it was evident that Sophia needed immediate advanced medical intervention.

Recognizing the gravity of the situation, the lead paramedic made a rapid decision. He pulled out his radio, his voice steady despite the severity of Sophia's condition, and called for a Life Flight helicopter.

The seconds ticked away, each one heavy with suspense as the team of paramedics tirelessly worked to preserve the life of the young girl. Soon, the rhythmic beat of helicopter blades slicing through the air became audible, a sound that heralded the Life Flight team. With precision, the helicopter descended rapidly, finding its landing spot in the closest available clearing.

Despite the helicopter, the paramedics remained focused on Sophia's well-being.

Sophia, still unresponsive, was carefully transferred from the ambulance onto the helicopter. The flight crew, consisting of a pilot, a nurse, and a paramedic, immediately got to work. Their faces were calm, focused, but their eyes reflected the magnitude of the situation.

The roar of the helicopter's rotor blades filled the small cabin as the Life Flight team hurried to stabilize two-year-old Sophia. She was suffering from severe heatstroke. The medical team worked with practiced precision, their hands steady despite the turbulence.

In an effort to lower Sophia's body temperature, the flight nurse softly placed a cool pack on her forehead and groin. Her tiny chest rose and fell rapidly, a testament to her body's fight against the heatstroke. An IV was inserted into her arm, delivering vital fluids to combat dehydration.

The paramedic conferred with the hospital via radio, providing real-time updates on Sophia's condition. The urgency in his voice was masked by the professional calmness he displayed, knowing that every second counted in this life-or-death situation.

Outside the window, the city lights were a blur, a stark contrast to the tense atmosphere inside the helicopter. The pilot navigated through the sky with a singular focus - to get Sophia to the hospital as quickly as possible.

As the helicopter neared its destination, the medical team prepared for landing, securing all loose items and double-checking Sophia's vitals.

Upon arrival, the academic hospital was already prepared for Sophia's arrival. The best pediatric specialists were on standby, ready to do everything in their power to save this young life. The Life Flight helicopter touched down on the hospital's rooftop helipad, its blades whirring to a stop as the medical team rushed Sophia into the emergency room. Their faces, etched with determination and worry, reflected the gravity of the situation.

This was not just any hospital. Renowned for its state-of-the-art facilities and world-class doctors, it was a prestigious medical institution where miracles were performed daily. Cutting-edge technology hummed quietly in the background, ready to assist the expert staff. The hospital's reputation as a beacon of hope drew patients from all corners of the globe, seeking solace and healing within its pristine walls.

Inside the emergency room, a team of expert doctors and nurses awaited Sophia's arrival. The air crackled with anticipation as they prepared to put their skills to the test. They had been briefed about her condition and were ready to employ every available resource to save her. The room buzzed with a sense of urgency as they began their lifesaving work, their every move a testament to their unwavering dedication.

They worked tirelessly, their hands moving with practiced ease as they administered treatment. Sophia, so small and fragile, put up a brave fight. The hours ticked by, turning into a night of endless waiting. Baby Sophia was transferred to the pediatric intensive care unit (PICU).

Despite the best efforts of the medical team, Sophia's condition remained critical. The heatstroke had caused significant damage, impairing her vital organs. The PICU staff worked around the clock, employing the latest interventions and treatments available in Pediatric Critical Care Medicine.

Days turned into weeks. Sophia fought bravely, showing signs of improvement at times, giving everyone a glimmer of hope. But the severity of her condition was too great, and her tiny body had endured too much.

One heartbreaking day, despite all the efforts, Sophia's vital signs began to worsen. The medical team entered with a sense of urgency, their expressions filled with tension as they tirelessly and persistently worked to rescue her. Nevertheless, the strain became too much for Sophia's little heart to handle.

With a heavy heart, the doctor had to deliver the devastating news to Sophia's parents. Sophia had succumbed to the complications related to the heatstroke.

Sophia's tragic loss deeply affected everyone, highlighting the deadly risks of leaving children in hot cars and underscoring the urgent need for increased awareness to prevent such incidents.

Leaving children in hot cars can be fatal. Each year, an average of 38 children under 15 die from heatstroke in vehicles. Children's bodies heat up faster, increasing the risk of heatstroke. These incidents can happen to anyone, even caring parents.

Rapid increase in temperature: Vehicles can heat up quickly, regardless of the outside temperature. Research shows that almost 53% of children who die from car-related heatstroke are left in the vehicle accidentally.

Children's ability to regulate temperature: Children and infants don't have as great of an ability to regulate their temperature, making it quite dangerous for them.

Potential for injury or death: Even the best of parents or caregivers can unknowingly leave a sleeping baby in a car, and the end result can be injury or even death.

Never leave a child unattended in a vehicle, not even for a minute.

Always lock your cars, even in your own driveway. Kids might play in cars or wander outside and get into a car.

Establish reminders: Place something you'll need at your next stop - like a briefcase or cell phone - next to the child safety seat. It can be easy to forget a quiet, sleeping infant in the back of a car.

If you encounter a child left in a hot car, call 911 immediately if the child seems hot or sick. If the child is unresponsive, do everything possible to get them out of the car, even if that means breaking a window.

THE UNSEEN ROAD AHEAD

In the heart of a crisp autumn day, the Moore family and their closest friends eagerly embarked on their cherished fall tradition—a delightful hayride through the golden-hued fields of their sprawling farm. The youngest, little Ellie, a spirited four-year-old, radiated excitement, her gleeful laughter harmonizing with the rustling leaves and the rhythmic chugging of the tractor.

Their trusty old tractor, driven by Mr. Moore's attentive gaze, pulled the wagon with a steady and comforting pace. The air was filled with the warm and picturesque glow of the sun, painting a scene of pure bliss and contentment as the group reveled in the joy of the moment. The path, though well-worn, was not without its hidden bumps and dips, a testament to the farm's rustic charm. Earlier, a minor jolt had elicited a chorus of laughter, a playful reminder of the tractor's age.

As they leisurely navigated the familiar path, Ellie and her family frolicked among the hay, their imaginations soaring as freely as the surrounding countryside. Yet, unbeknownst to them, a hidden danger lurked beneath the beauty of the moment—a deceptive dip in the road cleverly concealed by a thick carpet of fallen leaves.

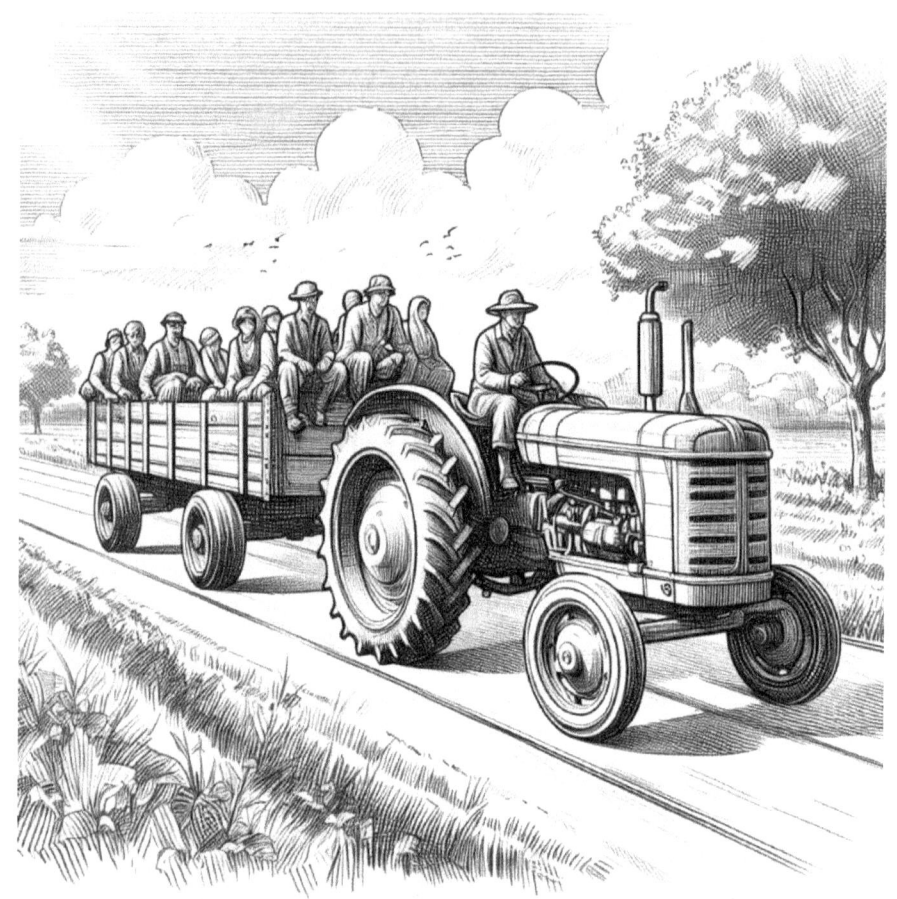

Suddenly, the wagon hit the unforeseen bump with a bone-jarring impact, sending shockwaves reverberating through the wooden frame. In a split second of chaos, Ellie was catapulted from the wagon, eliciting heart-wrenching cries of terror from her family and friends. As Mr. Moore attempted to stop the wagon, its wheel ominously approached her fallen form as they watched helplessly, the wheel rolled over Ellie's head with a sickening thud, shattering the tranquility of the moment. The world seemed to freeze in that horrifying instant, as gasps of horror filled the air and a grim reality set in.

Mr. Moore immediately understood the severity of the incident. He urgently stopped the tractor and called 911, his voice filled with concern as he described the situation. While help was on its way, Mr. Moore and the other family members did their best to take care of Ellie.

The Emergency Medical Services (EMS) team, clad in their distinctive uniforms, arrived promptly, their expertise evident in the swift and synchronized manner in which they assessed the emergency. Realizing the seriousness of the situation, they promptly mobilized and coordinated a Life Flight helicopter.

For Amy, the flight nurse aboard the rescue helicopter, each mission was a testament to the fragility and resilience of human life. As they approached the Moore family's location, she double-checked her medical supplies, knowing that every second would count upon their arrival. The helicopter's descent was swift, its blades slicing through the evening air with precision, as Amy and her team prepared to deploy. From her perspective, the mission was clear, yet fraught with the unknown–to stabilize and transport Ellie to the nearest Trauma Center as efficiently and safely as possible.

Upon landing, Amy was the first to disembark the helicopter, her steps quick and sure as she approached the scene. Her eyes, trained to assess in an instant, took in the sight of the distressed family and the small, still form of Ellie. Showing a composed and professional demeanor, Amy knelt down beside Ellie, providing words of comfort as she meticulously performed her important duties. Ellie's minimal response and shallow breaths indicated her imminent deterioration. Upon realizing the seriousness of Ellie's condition, Amy decided to place a breathing tube to ensure Ellie's airway was protected and she received the necessary oxygen to survive.

With practiced precision, Amy prepared the necessary equipment, her hands moving deftly as she selected the appropriate sized breathing tube and laryngoscope. Gently, she tilted Ellie's head back, visualizing the small opening of her airway. With a steady hand, she inserted the laryngoscope blade, expertly maneuvering it to reveal the vocal cords. In a moment of focused concentration, she skillfully guided the breathing tube through the vocal cords and into the trachea, ensuring its proper placement. The rhythmic whoosh of the ventilator filled the air as it began to breathe for Ellie, a reassuring sound amidst the chaos.

The transport back was tense, every minute a fight against time, but Amy's focus never wavered. Inside the helicopter, amidst the roar of the engines, a bubble of concentrated calm formed around her and her patient, as she worked to ensure Ellie's stability. This was more than a flight; it was a lifeline, and for Amy, it was a reminder of why she had chosen this path.

Throughout the journey, Amy's team worked in perfect unison, their individual skills merging into a seamless effort to save Ellie's life. As she monitored and adjusted medication and oxygen levels, her colleagues maintained communication with the hospital they were headed towards. They navigated through the sky, never losing sight of their goal – to deliver Ellie safely into the hands of skilled medical professionals. As the helicopter finally touched down at the hospital, Amy could breathe a small sigh of relief. Their mission was accomplished, and all that remained was for Ellie to receive the care she needed.

The outcome, while a testament to the skill and dedication of Amy and her team, was bittersweet. Ellie survived the harrowing ordeal thanks to their efforts, but the irreversible effects of her condition left her with permanent brain damage. The road ahead would be challenging, with adjustment and rehabilitation efforts tailored to help Ellie adapt to a new way of living. Her family, while relieved at her survival, faced the reality of her condition with a mixture of gratitude for the present and apprehension for the future. Support from healthcare professionals, love from her family, and a resilient spirit would now be Ellie's guiding lights as she navigated through her altered landscape of life.

Take Home Points

Going on a hayride can be a fantastic family activity, especially during the fall season! It's a great way to enjoy the outdoors and get a taste of farm life. However, it's important to keep safety in mind to ensure everyone has a good time with no mishaps. Here are some simplified tips geared towards families planning to go on a hayride:

Hold on to small children: Small children can be particularly vulnerable on hayrides because of unexpected bumps or sudden movements. It's important to always keep them securely in your lap or by your side. If the wagon hits a bump, small children could be thrown off if they're not held onto. Always make sure they're seated safely away from the edges and maintain a firm grip on them throughout the ride to prevent any accidents.

Stay seated properly: Once you find your spot on the hayride, stay seated with your arms and legs inside the wagon. The hay might be more slippery than you expect, so it's best to remain seated throughout the ride.

Follow the rules: Pay attention to any rules posted or given by the hayride operators. This includes listening to the attendants and not standing up during the ride. These rules are there to keep everyone safe.

Inspect the ride: If possible, look at the hay wagon and tractor before the ride starts. Check for anything that looks unsafe or out of place. Operators should inspect the equipment daily, but an extra set of eyes doesn't hurt.

Be careful when loading and unloading: Make sure to load and unload one person at a time. Adults should help children get on and off the ride safely. Avoid walking on the hay bales and stay seated unless you're getting off the ride.

Choose a safe route: If you have the opportunity, ask about the route the hayride will take. It's best to avoid major roads and choose a path that's away from traffic and other hazards. A smoother, less trafficked route makes for a safer and more enjoyable ride.

Families can have a safe and enjoyable hayride experience by following these easy tips.

LOCKED OUT IN THE COLD

An unexpected turn of events shattered the cozy warmth of the Smith family home on a cold winter morning. In the middle of the night, Little Mason, a curious four-year-old, began to explore his house as his parents slept. As he wandered through the living room, he noticed the snow outside the front door, beckoning him to the winter wonderland outside.

Mason, fascinated by the glistening snow, cautiously opened the door, and stepped onto the porch. The crisp air sent shivers down his spine, but the allure of the snow-covered yard was too strong to resist. He closed the door behind him, unaware that the lock had clicked shut, trapping him outside in the freezing cold.

Mason's initial excitement quickly turned to fear as he realized he couldn't get back inside. He pounded on the door, his tiny hands numb from the cold, but his cries went unheard. His parents were still fast asleep, oblivious to their son's predicament.

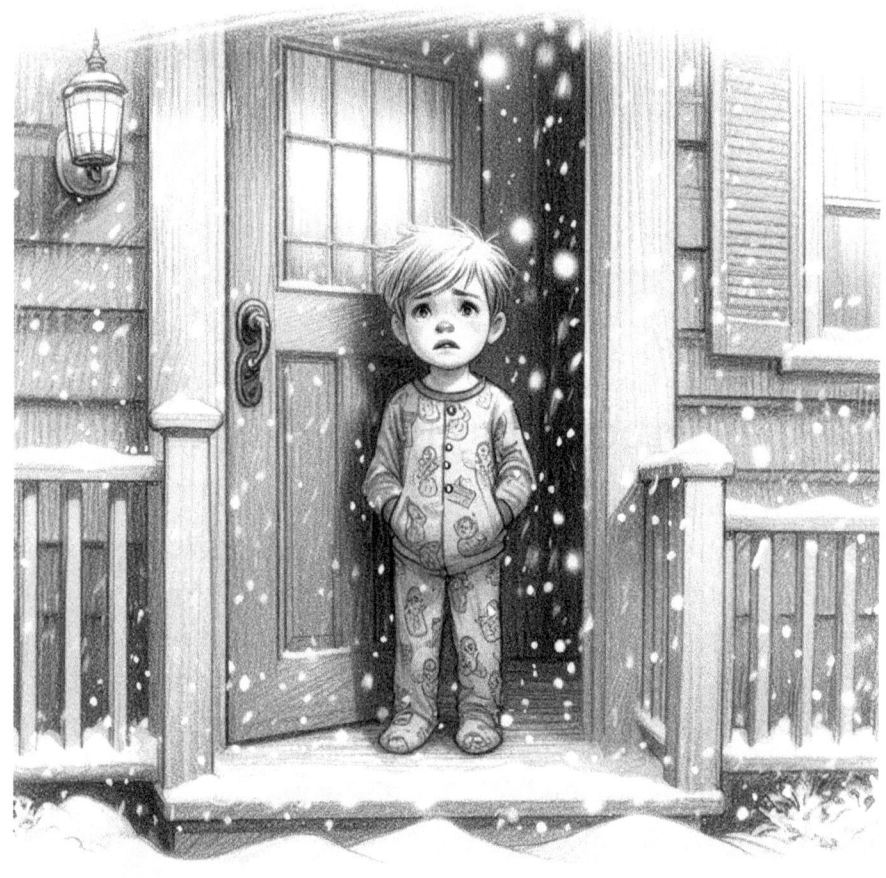

The winter wind howled, chilling Mason to the bone. He huddled on the porch, tears streaming down his cheeks, his little body shivering uncontrollably. He longed for the warmth of his home, the comfort of his parents' embrace.

As the minutes turned into what felt like hours, Mason's cries grew weaker, his energy fading. He curled up in a ball, hoping to conserve whatever warmth remained in his tiny frame. The snow continued to fall, blanketing him in a cold, white embrace.

Just as Mason's consciousness began to slip away, his mother awoke, startled by the silence in the house. She looked around for Mason but couldn't find him anywhere. Panic set in as she realized he wasn't in his bed or any of his usual hiding spots. A frantic search ensued, and as she peered out the window, she saw a small figure huddled on the porch, covered in snow.

She felt a sudden surge of adrenaline as she rushed to the door, fumbling with the lock. Finally, she opened it and scooped up her shivering son, tears of relief streaming down her face. Every second felt like an eternity as she held him close, his tiny body limp in her arms.

Overcome with a mix of relief and terror, she rushed back inside, Mason's ice-cold skin and blue lips a stark reminder of the severity of the situation. Without hesitation, she dialed 911, her voice trembling as she explained the situation to the dispatcher. The urgency in her tone was palpable, and the dispatcher assured her that help was on the way. The distant wail of sirens, a sound both terrifying and reassuring, finally broke the morning silence.

Within minutes, an ambulance pulled into the Smith's driveway. Paramedics rushed into the house, their faces etched with concern as they assessed Mason's condition. They worked quickly, administering oxygen and starting an IV to deliver warm fluids.

Mason's core temperature remained dangerously cold despite the paramedics' efforts. Recognizing the severity of his hypothermia and the specialized care he urgently needed, they made the critical decision to call for a Life Flight. The nearest children's hospital with advanced warming capabilities was over 50 miles away, and with Mason's life hanging in the balance, every minute counted.

A helicopter soon landed in a nearby field, its rotors whipping up a flurry of snow. Mason, still in critical condition, was carefully transferred to the helicopter, his parents watching with tear-filled eyes as their precious son was airlifted to the hospital.

The flight was intense, with each second seeming like an eternity. The medical team onboard worked tirelessly, monitoring Mason's vitals, and providing continuous care. Back at their house, his parents anxiously began the drive to the hospital, their hearts heavy with guilt and worry, praying for their son's survival.

Upon arrival at the hospital, Mason was immediately rushed to the emergency room, where a team of specialists was waiting. He was placed in a warming blanket, and a series of tests were conducted to assess the extent of the damage caused by the hypothermia.

The following hours were agonizing for the Smith family. They waited anxiously for any news, their hopes and fears battling within them. Finally, a doctor emerged, his expression grave but with a glimmer of hope. Mason's condition was critical, but he was responding to treatment. He had a long road to recovery ahead, but he was a fighter.

Mason was admitted to the pediatric intensive care unit (PICU), where a team of specialists closely monitored him. His core body temperature had dropped dangerously low, and the doctors worked tirelessly to gradually rewarm him. They used warming blankets, warm intravenous fluids, and even a special machine that circulated warm air around his body.

The hypothermia had wreaked havoc on Mason's small body. His heart struggled to maintain a steady rhythm, his breaths came in short, shallow gasps, and his blood pressure had dropped alarmingly low. The doctors administered medications to stabilize his faltering vital signs, working to prevent the dangerous cascade of complications that could arise from his prolonged exposure to the cold.

Mason's parents remained by his side, their hearts heavy with worry. They watched as the doctors and nurses worked tirelessly to save their son's life. The hours turned into days, and Mason's condition slowly but steadily improved.

After several days in the PICU, Mason was finally stable enough to be transferred to a regular hospital room. He was still weak and required ongoing care, but he was on the road to recovery. His parents were overjoyed to see their son's progress, and they were grateful for the skilled and compassionate care he had received.

Mason's struggle was a chilling occurrence, but it led his parents to understand their complacency about childproofing their home. They vowed to make changes to prevent such an incident from happening again. Childproof locks were installed on all exterior doors, ensuring they were out of Mason's reach and only operable by adults. They added door alarms that would sound if a door was opened, providing an immediate alert if Mason attempted to venture outside unnoticed.

Window locks were a priority. His parents installed childproof window guards that allowed for ventilation but prevented windows from being opened wide enough for a child to slip through. They moved furniture away from windows to eliminate potential climbing aids.

Realizing that Mason's curiosity extended beyond doors and windows, they embarked on a thorough childproofing mission throughout the house. Electrical outlets were covered with safety plugs, sharp corners were cushioned, and hazardous substances were stored in locked cabinets well out of Mason's reach. They installed a baby gate at the top of the stairs to prevent any accidental falls, and they secured heavy furniture and appliances to the wall to avoid tip-overs.

Beyond physical safeguards, his parents focused on educating Mason about safety. The dangers of going outside alone, especially in cold weather, were taught to him, and he was strongly advised to always inform an adult before leaving the house. They used age-appropriate books and videos to reinforce these messages and engaged him in interactive safety games to make learning fun.

A well-defined and consistent routine was implemented for bedtime and outdoor play, giving Mason a sense of security and clear boundaries. They created a designated play area in the backyard, equipped with safe and engaging toys, and always supervised him when he was playing outside.

The Smith family's journey towards childproofing their home was an ongoing process, one that required constant vigilance and adaptation as Mason grew and developed. Through their efforts, they created a safer environment for their son, one where he could explore and learn without putting himself in harm's way.

Mason's frightening experience serves as a powerful reminder of the dangers of hypothermia and the critical importance of prevention and swift action. Parents can safeguard their children and prevent similar incidents by adopting some fundamental safety practices. These include installing childproof locks and doorknob covers, educating children about the risks of venturing outside alone, particularly during inclement weather, and regularly inspecting doors and windows for security.

It's vital to maintain close supervision of young children, especially near potential exits. In the unfortunate event that a child gets locked out in the cold, immediate action is crucial. Bring them inside without delay, remove wet clothing, and wrap them in warm blankets. If conscious and able to swallow, offer warm liquids.

Seek medical attention promptly, even if the child appears fine, and equip yourself with CPR and basic first aid skills for children. These preventative measures and emergency responses can make all the difference in protecting our little ones from the harsh elements and ensuring their safety.

Here are some additional tips for preventing children from accidentally locking themselves out:

Door alarms: Install door alarms that sound when a door is opened. This can alert you if a child is trying to go outside unsupervised.

Door chains: Install door chains high up on the door where children can't reach them. This allows you to open the door slightly for ventilation while keeping it securely closed.

Supervision: When expecting deliveries or visitors, ensure young children are supervised or in a secure area away from the door to prevent them from slipping out unnoticed.

Practice drills: Conduct practice drills with your children, teaching them what to do if they accidentally get locked out. This could include staying near the door, calling for help, or going to a trusted neighbor's house.

Remember, childproofing is an ongoing process as children grow and become more curious. Regularly assess your home for potential risks and adjust your safety measures accordingly.

LILY'S TUMBLE

The sun glowed through the kitchen window as two-year-old Lily played on the living room floor. Her tiny hands expertly maneuvered a dollhouse, her imagination filling the space with lively conversations between the miniature inhabitants. Her grandmother, humming a soft tune, was busy preparing lunch, occasionally glancing over to check on her granddaughter. The house was filled with the comforting sounds of everyday life.

Suddenly, a sharp cry pierced the air, followed by a loud thud. Grandma's heart skipped a beat as she rushed towards the sound. The latch to the basement door, which Lily had managed to open, was not secured.

Grandma rushed down the stairs to Lily's side, her heart pounding in her chest. The little girl was pale and unresponsive, a thin line of blood trickling from her forehead. Panic surged through Grandma, but she forced herself to stay calm. She carefully scooped Lily into her arms, cradling her close to her chest. With trembling hands, she dialed 911, her voice barely above a whisper as she relayed the terrifying details to the dispatcher.

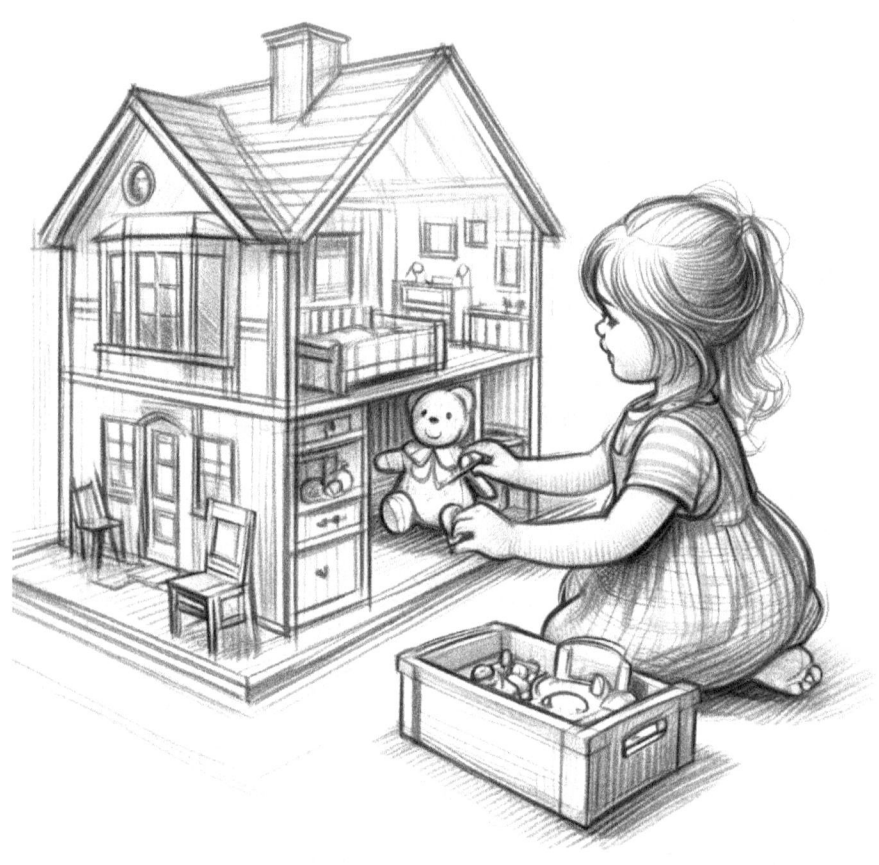

The minutes felt like hours as Grandma anxiously awaited the paramedics. She paced the living room floor, her mind racing with a million thoughts. What if Lily was seriously hurt? What if she had suffered permanent damage? Guilt gnawed at her – she should have been watching Lily more closely. She should have installed a child safety gate at the top of the stairs.

The sound of sirens approaching brought Grandma back to the present. The paramedics burst through the front door, their faces etched with a mixture of concern and determination. They quickly assessed Lily's condition, their movements efficient and practiced. One paramedic gently lifted Lily from

Grandma's arms, while another began attaching monitoring equipment.

The living room was transformed into a makeshift emergency room, with the paramedics working swiftly to stabilize Lily. They started an IV, administered medications, and carefully immobilized her neck. Grandma watched helplessly, her heart aching as she saw her precious granddaughter lying so still and pale.

The paramedics spoke in hushed tones, their words a blur to Grandma's ears. She caught snippets of their conversation – "head injury," "possible fracture," "need for transport." Her anxiety grew with each passing minute.

Finally, one of the paramedics approached Grandma, his expression grave. "We need to transport Lily to a Trauma Center in the city," he explained. "Her injuries are serious, and she needs specialized care." Grandma nodded, her eyes filling with tears. She knew this was the best course of action, but the thought of Lily being airlifted away filled her with dread.

The paramedic continued, "We've called for a Life Flight helicopter. It will meet us at the nearby rendezvous site." Grandma watched as the paramedics carefully moved Lily to the ambulance, securing her to a stretcher and covering her with a warm blanket.

The ambulance sped off, its sirens wailing, as Grandma followed closely behind in her car. Her mind raced with worry and fear for her granddaughter's safety. As they approached the rendezvous site, Grandma could see the helicopter circling overhead, its powerful blades slicing through the air.

The helicopter arrived, its rotors kicking up a whirlwind of dust and debris as it touched down on the helipad. The flight nurse, Riley, and the flight paramedic, Tom, worked quickly and efficiently to transfer Lily from the ambulance stretcher to the helicopter's specialized stretcher. They secured her tiny body with straps, ensuring she was safe and stable for the flight.

The cabin was cramped, yet the tension that permeated the space was somehow kept under control. The sound of the rotors created a rhythmic thumping in the air. Riley and Tom, nevertheless, stayed cool and concentrated, their years of experience evident in their every move.

Riley expertly managed Lily's airway, ensuring she was receiving adequate oxygen. She monitored the little girl's vital signs, noting with concern her rapid heart rate and shallow breathing. As Lily's level of consciousness continued to decrease, Riley made the difficult decision to insert a breathing tube to protect her airway and ensure proper ventilation.

Tom, meanwhile, prepared medications and fluids, ready to administer them at a moment's notice. He assisted Riley with the intubation, their movements precise and coordinated despite the cramped quarters and the deafening noise of the rotors.

Throughout the flight, Riley and Tom communicated constantly, updating each other on Lily's condition and adjusting their treatment plan as needed. They worked seamlessly as a team, their primary focus keeping Lily alive and stable until they reached the Trauma Center.

The flight was bumpy, and the helicopter swayed with every gust of wind. But Riley and Tom never wavered in their care for Lily. They spoke to her in soothing tones, offering words of comfort even though she remained unconscious.

As the helicopter approached the city, the skyline came into view, its towering buildings a stark contrast to the rural landscape they had left behind. Riley radioed ahead to the Trauma Center, providing an update on Lily's condition and estimated time of arrival.

The helicopter landed smoothly on the hospital's rooftop helipad, and a team of medical professionals was waiting to receive Lily. Riley and Tom carefully transferred her to a waiting stretcher, their faces etched with fatigue but also with a sense of accomplishment. They had done their part, and now it was up to the trauma team to continue the fight for Lily's life.

Upon arrival at the Trauma Center, Lily was rushed into surgery. The trauma surgeon made a skillful attempt to repair and minimize damage, working meticulously to prevent additional complications. The surgery was a success, but Lily's journey was far from over. She was then transferred to the pediatric intensive care unit, where a team of specialized doctors and nurses closely monitored her condition.

Days turned into weeks as Lily slowly regained consciousness. Her recovery was marked by small victories and occasional setbacks. There were moments of clarity when she would recognize her parents and respond to their voices, followed by periods of confusion and disorientation. The medical team explained that this was a normal part of the healing process, but it was still difficult for Lily's family to witness.

Lily's parents remained by her side day and night, their hearts filled with a mixture of hope and fear. They celebrated every milestone, no matter how small – a squeeze of the hand, a flicker of recognition in her eyes. They also endured the moments when Lily seemed to regress, her progress halted by the severity of her injuries.

As the weeks passed, Lily gradually regained her strength and mobility. Physical therapists worked with her tirelessly, helping her to relearn basic movements and coordination. Speech therapists helped her to regain her ability to communicate, and occupational therapists assisted her with everyday tasks.

The fall had left its mark. Lily had suffered some permanent damage to her motor skills, and she would walk with a slight limp for the rest of her life. However, her cognitive abilities remained intact, and her spirit was as bright and vibrant as ever.

The accident had a profound impact on the relationship between Lily's parents and her grandmother. Initially, feelings of guilt and blame cast a shadow over their interactions. Lily's parents, while grateful for their mother's love and care for Lily, couldn't help but harbor some resentment over the incident. The grandmother, already burdened by guilt, felt their unspoken accusations keenly.

However, as Lily's condition improved, they slowly began to heal together. Recognizing their shared love for Lily, they chose to focus on her recovery rather than dwelling on the past. Open communication and understanding gradually replaced the initial tension, and their bond grew stronger through the shared experience.

With the help of dedicated therapists and the unwavering support of her family, Lily continued to make progress. Once again, her laughter echoed through the air as she relearned to walk, navigate obstacles, and enjoy playtime. Her resilience was an inspiration to everyone who knew her, and her family's love and encouragement helped her to overcome every obstacle.

Lily's parents were committed to providing her with the best possible care and support as she continued her recovery at home. They worked closely with the medical team to develop a comprehensive plan that addressed Lily's physical, emotional, and cognitive needs.

To ensure Lily's safety and facilitate her mobility, several adjustments were made to their home. Stair gates were installed at the top and bottom of every staircase, and non-slip mats were placed in the bathrooms and kitchen. Furniture was rearranged to create clear pathways, and potential hazards were removed.

Lily's parents also received training from the therapists to continue her rehabilitation exercises at home. They learned how to assist her with daily activities, such as dressing, bathing, and eating, while encouraging her independence as much as possible. They also implemented strategies to manage any emotional or behavioral challenges that might arise as Lily adjusted to her new limitations.

In addition to the physical adjustments and therapeutic exercises, Lily's parents recognized the importance of emotional support and open communication. They created a safe and nurturing environment where Lily felt comfortable expressing her feelings and concerns. They also sought out support groups and counseling services to help them navigate the challenges of caring for a child with a disability.

Lily's story highlights the need for proactive measures to prevent stair accidents, particularly for curious and adventurous young children. Here are some essential tips:

Install safety gates: Use sturdy safety gates at the top and bottom of staircases to prevent young children from accessing them unsupervised. Choose gates that are specifically designed for stair use and that meet current safety standards. Ensure they are securely installed and cannot be easily dislodged by a child.

Secure carpets and rugs: Prevent slips and trips by securing rugs with non-slip pads or double-sided tape. Regularly check for any curled edges or loose areas and repair or replace as needed. Consider using carpet runners with non-slip backing on hardwood or tile floors.

Supervise young children: Never leave a young child unattended near stairs or other potential hazards. Even if you think your child is old enough to navigate stairs safely, accidents can happen in a split second. Direct supervision is crucial, especially for toddlers and younger children.

Teach stair safety: As soon as they are old enough, teach children how to climb stairs safely, emphasizing the importance of holding onto the railing and taking one step at a time. Make it a fun and engaging activity, using songs or games to reinforce the message.

Keep stairs clutter-free: Remove any toys, shoes, or other objects that could obstruct the stairs and create a tripping hazard. Ensure that the stairs are well-lit and free of any spills or slippery substances.

Regularly inspect your home: Conduct routine safety checks of your home, paying close attention to areas where falls are more likely to occur. This includes not only stairs but also balconies, windows, and high furniture.

Be prepared for emergencies: Keep a first-aid kit readily available and know how to administer basic first aid for injuries such as cuts, bruises, and head injuries. In case of a serious fall, call 911 immediately and provide clear and concise information about the situation.

By following these simple precautions, we can help protect our children and prevent devastating accidents like Lily's. Remember, a few moments of prevention can make a lifetime of difference.

A MOTHER'S NIGHTMARE

Aubrey, a young mother, was enjoying a warm spring afternoon in her backyard with her three-year-old son, Alex. Laughter filled the air as Alex chased butterflies, his small feet padding softly across the lush green lawn. The sweet scent of blooming flowers hung heavy in the air, and a gentle breeze rustled the leaves of the trees that lined the property. Aubrey, momentarily distracted by a phone call, glanced away from her son, her attention divided between the conversation and keeping a watchful eye on Alex.

Their backyard was enclosed by a tall, sturdy fence, creating a seemingly safe haven for Alex to play. However, nestled in a far corner of the property, hidden from view by a cluster of flowering shrubs, a small gate leading to a nearby pond remained unlocked—a detail that would soon shatter their peaceful afternoon.

Drawn by the allure of the shimmering water, Alex wandered toward the gate, his curiosity outweighing any sense of caution. Engrossed in her conversation, Aubrey didn't notice her son slip away until an eerie silence fell over the yard.

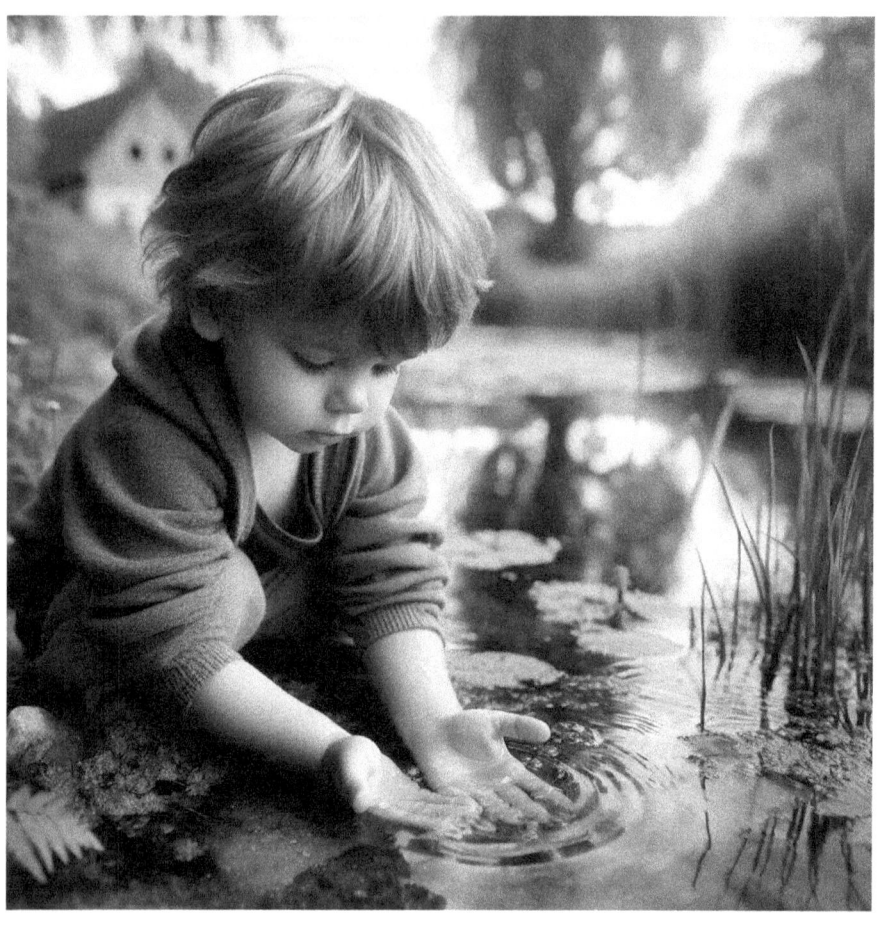

Panic surged through Aubrey as she frantically scanned the yard, her heart pounding in her chest. Spotting the open gate and the pond beyond, a wave of dread washed over her. She raced toward the water, her mind filled with a mother's worst nightmare.

Reaching the pond's edge, Aubrey's heart sank. Alex's small, lifeless body floated face down in the murky depths. With a cry of anguish, she plunged in, pulling him to shore. His skin was cold, his lips blue, his eyes closed.

Aubrey's instincts kicked in. She desperately performed CPR, her breath shallow, her hands trembling. Time seemed to stand still as she fought to save her son. Realizing the severity of the situation, she screamed for help, her voice echoing across the still water. Two neighbors rushed to her aid, one of them immediately calling 911 while another assisted Aubrey with CPR.

The sound of sirens grew louder as paramedics arrived. They quickly took over, their grim expressions mirroring the seriousness of the matter. Despite their continuous CPR attempts, little Alex could not be revived, and the Emergency Medical Services (EMS) crew continued CPR throughout the journey to the hospital.

Anticipating the severity of Alex's condition ahead of time, they had already made arrangements for a Life Flight helicopter to rendezvous with them. The nearest pediatric intensive care unit was over an hour away by ambulance, and every second was critical.

The helicopter touched down at the small hospital near Aubrey's home not long after the EMS crew arrived. After several more minutes of CPR, the medical teams were able to obtain a pulse shortly after inserting a breathing tube into Alex's small trachea. They considered taking little Alex inside the small hospital but knew his best chance would be a transfer to a large academic medical center.

Both teams swiftly moved Alex onto a stretcher and into the aircraft. Inside the cramped, noisy cabin, Natalie, a seasoned flight nurse with years of experience, took charge.

The atmosphere was tense. The rhythmic thumping of the helicopter blades, the constant beeping of monitors, and the urgent chatter of the medical team created a sense of controlled chaos. Natalie, however, remained calm and focused.

She carefully assessed Alex, checking his vital signs, and adjusting the settings on the ventilator that breathed for him. His heart rate was weak, his blood pressure dangerously low. Natalie understood that they were in a race against time.

As the helicopter rose, the surroundings became blurred underneath them. Natalie's mind raced, going over the steps she needed to take to stabilize Alex's condition. She administered medications to support his heart and lungs, her hands moving with practiced precision.

Minutes felt like hours as Natalie and her team worked tirelessly. The inside of the helicopter, illuminated by medical equipment, had a mix of claustrophobic and oddly comforting vibes. It was a place where the equilibrium of life and death was fragile, and where every action could determine the outcome between surviving and experiencing tragedy.

Upon arrival at the hospital, Alex was immediately rushed to the pediatric intensive care unit (PICU). The medical team, a well-coordinated orchestra of doctors, nurses, and specialists, worked tirelessly to stabilize his condition. They monitored his vital signs, administered medications, and performed a battery of tests to assess the extent of the damage. Aubrey, a silent observer in this whirlwind of activity, could only watch and pray, her heart aching with every beep of the machines and every whispered consultation.

As the hours turned into days, Alex's condition remained critical but stable. He was placed in a medically induced coma to allow his body to rest and heal. The ventilator breathed for him, and a feeding tube provided him with essential nutrients. The doctors explained to Aubrey that the next few days would be crucial, as they closely monitored his brain activity and neurological function.

Despite the medical team's best efforts, the damage to Alex's brain was irreversible. The prolonged lack of oxygen had resulted in severe neurological impairment, leaving him in a persistent vegetative state. He would never regain consciousness, never experience the world around him, never fulfill the potential that had once sparkled in his bright eyes.

The news shattered Aubrey's world. She had held onto a glimmer of hope, a desperate belief that her son would somehow defy the odds. Now, faced with the harsh reality of his condition, she felt a profound sense of loss and despair.

Aubrey was devastated, consumed by guilt and grief. She replayed the events of that afternoon, blaming herself for the tragedy. She had lost the son she knew, and the future she had envisioned for him.

In the aftermath, Aubrey became an advocate for water safety, sharing her story to prevent other families from experiencing the same heartbreak. She dedicated her life to caring for Alex, ensuring he received the best possible care and therapy.

Drowning is a leading cause of death for young children and can occur in seconds, even in shallow water. Constant supervision is essential around pools, ponds, and any body of water, as a momentary distraction can have devastating consequences. Preventive measures for drowning involve:

Install fences: Ensure pools and other bodies of water are enclosed with fences that have self-closing, self-latching gates to prevent unsupervised access.

Teach water safety: Educate children on basic water safety skills, such as floating, treading water, and the dangers of water.

Swimming lessons: Enroll children in swimming lessons to enhance their water competency and confidence.

Supervise vigilantly: Always keep a close watch on children in or around water, regardless of their swimming abilities. Designate a "water watcher" to maintain undistracted supervision.

Learn CPR: Acquire CPR and basic first aid skills to be prepared for emergencies. Knowing how to respond quickly can save lives.

Use life jackets: Ensure children wear life jackets when boating or near open water, even if they know how to swim.

Remove toys from pools: After swimming, remove toys from the pool area to prevent children from being tempted to reach for them and accidentally falling in.

Educate on pool drains: Teach children to avoid pool drains and suction outlets to prevent entrapment.

BREATHLESS BITE

In a cozy suburban home, a loving father named Mark was preparing dinner while his 8-year-old daughter, Leah, sat at the kitchen table, excitedly chatting about her day at school. The aroma of freshly baked bread filled the air, and the sound of Leah's laughter brought a warm smile to Mark's face. As he placed a plate of sliced apples in front of her, Leah reached for a piece, her eyes sparkling with joy.

Suddenly, a look of panic crossed Leah's face as she began to cough violently. Mark rushed to her side, patting her back gently, but the coughing only intensified. Leah's face turned red, and her eyes began to bulge as she struggled to breathe.

Mark, terrified and unsure of what to do, tried to remain calm. He tried to give Leah water, hoping it would dislodge whatever was stuck in her throat, but she couldn't swallow. As Leah's condition rapidly deteriorated, Mark's panic grew. He didn't know how to perform the Heimlich maneuver, and precious seconds slipped away.

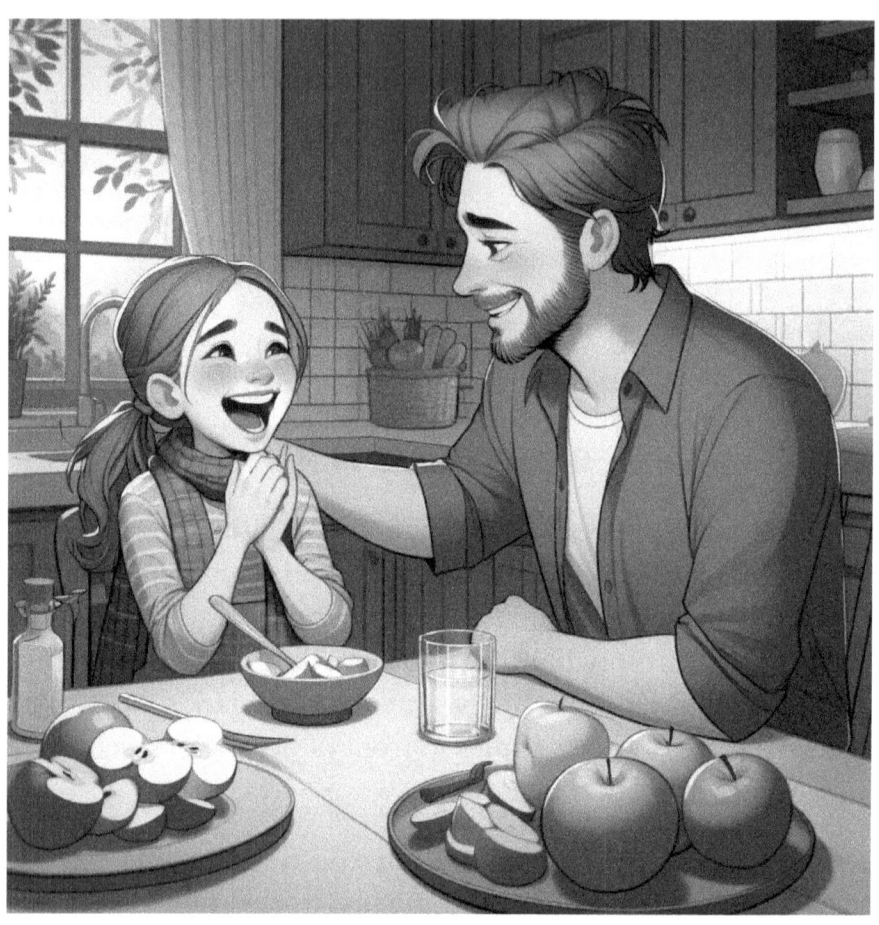

Understanding the severity of the situation, Mark frantically called 911. The dispatcher, sensing the urgency in his voice, calmly guided him through the steps of the Heimlich maneuver while an ambulance was dispatched to their home.

The paramedics arrived within minutes and found Leah unconscious and unresponsive. They quickly took over, performing the Heimlich maneuver and successfully dislodging the piece of apple that had been blocking her airway. However, Leah remained unconscious, and her breathing was shallow and labored.

The paramedics immediately began to support her breathing with advanced life support measures, working tirelessly to revive her. Despite their best efforts, Leah's condition did not improve. Knowing that Leah needed specialized care, the paramedics called for a Life Flight helicopter to transport her to a nearby medical center with a dedicated pediatric intensive care unit.

As the helicopter landed in a nearby field, the medical team swiftly transferred Leah to a stretcher and into the aircraft. Inside the cramped interior, a seasoned flight nurse named Lisa took charge.

Knowing that Leah was unconscious and struggling to breathe, Lisa made the critical decision to intubate her before they even left the ground. With practiced efficiency, she skillfully inserted a breathing tube into Leah's airway, securing it in place. This would ensure that Leah received the necessary oxygen and ventilation support during the flight to the hospital.

After ensuring that the airway was secured, Lisa gave the pilot the green light to start up the aircraft and depart from the scene. The atmosphere was tense. The steady thumping of the helicopter blades and the urgent chatter of the medical team gave the impression of organized chaos. Lisa, nonetheless, stayed calm and focused, her years of experience guiding her through the crisis.

Now that Leah's airway was secured, Lisa turned her attention to the ventilator, carefully adjusting the settings to provide the optimal support for Leah's breathing.

As the helicopter lifted off, the landscape blurred beneath them. Lisa's brain hurriedly processed the steps she needed to take to stabilize Leah's condition. She administered medications to support her cardiovascular and respiratory systems, her hands moving with practiced precision.

Lisa and her team dedicated themselves to supporting and closely monitoring Leah's critical condition, and each passing minute seemed to stretch into hours. The helicopter's interior, bathed in the eerie glow of medical equipment, felt both claustrophobic and strangely comforting. It was a place where the line between life and death was delicate, and where every action could determine the distinction between survival and tragedy.

Upon arrival at the hospital, Leah was rushed into the pediatric intensive care unit. A team of specialists worked tirelessly to save her life. After what felt like an eternity, Leah's eyes slowly fluttered open. She was weak and confused, but she was alive. The medical team was overjoyed, and Leah's parents were overwhelmed with relief.

Leah's recovery was long and difficult, but she was a fighter. With the support of her family and the dedicated medical staff, she slowly regained her strength and cognitive abilities. After weeks of intensive therapy and rehabilitation, Leah was finally able to go home.

Her homecoming was a joyous occasion, filled with laughter, tears, and a renewed appreciation for life. Leah's near-death experience had a profound impact on her and her family, teaching them the preciousness of every moment and the importance of cherishing the loved ones around them.

Mark became an advocate for first aid and CPR training, sharing his story to raise awareness about the importance of knowing how to respond in a choking emergency. He dedicated his life to ensuring that other parents would have the knowledge and skills to save their children's lives.

Take Home Points

Choking occurs when an object, such as food or a small item, becomes lodged in the throat or windpipe, blocking the flow of air. This blockage prevents oxygen from reaching the lungs and brain, which can quickly become life-threatening. In adults, choking is often caused by food, while young children may choke on small objects they put in their mouths.

When the airway is partially blocked, the person may cough forcefully in an attempt to dislodge the object. However, if the airway is completely blocked, the person cannot breathe, speak, or cough, and may show the universal sign of choking: clutching their throat with one or both hands. Immediate action is crucial to prevent suffocation and potential brain damage due to lack of oxygen.

Having the skill to perform the Heimlich maneuver can mean the difference between life and death in a choking emergency. To prevent choking, it is essential to cut food into small, manageable pieces for young children, supervise them while they are eating, and encourage them to eat slowly and chew their food thoroughly. Additionally, avoiding hard, round foods like nuts, grapes, and popcorn for young children can reduce the risk of choking. Learning CPR and basic first aid for children is also crucial. By following these safety measures and acquiring basic first aid skills, we can help prevent choking and protect our children from harm.

Universal Choking Sign

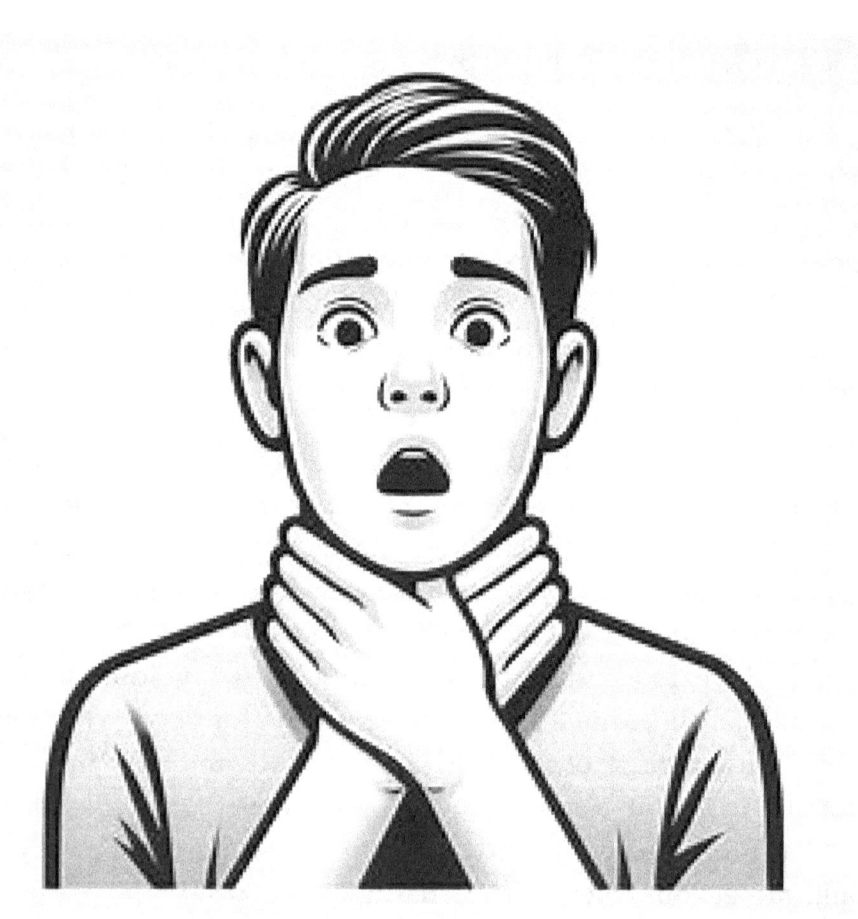

A HERO THAT MADE A DIFFERENCE

The sun-drenched November afternoon painted a stark contrast to the week of relentless rain, casting a deceptive golden glow over the landscape. The air, crisp and cool, carried the scent of damp earth and fallen leaves, a poignant reminder of the fleeting beauty of autumn. As 14-year-old Samantha embarked on an All-Terrain Vehicle (ATV) ride with her friends, Sarah and Mike, the world seemed to hold its breath, the vibrant hues of the forest masking the lurking danger.

Their laughter echoed through the towering trees, momentarily drowning out the rumble of the ATV engine. The familiar path wound its way through the woods, a comforting rhythm of twists and turns. But as they approached a sharp bend, a moment of distraction, a split-second loss of control, shattered the tranquility.

The ATV deviated from its course, its tires skidding on the slick leaves. The world tilted, a kaleidoscope of greens and browns blurring into a chaotic frenzy. And then, with a sickening crunch, the ATV collided with an ancient oak, its gnarled branches reaching out like skeletal arms.

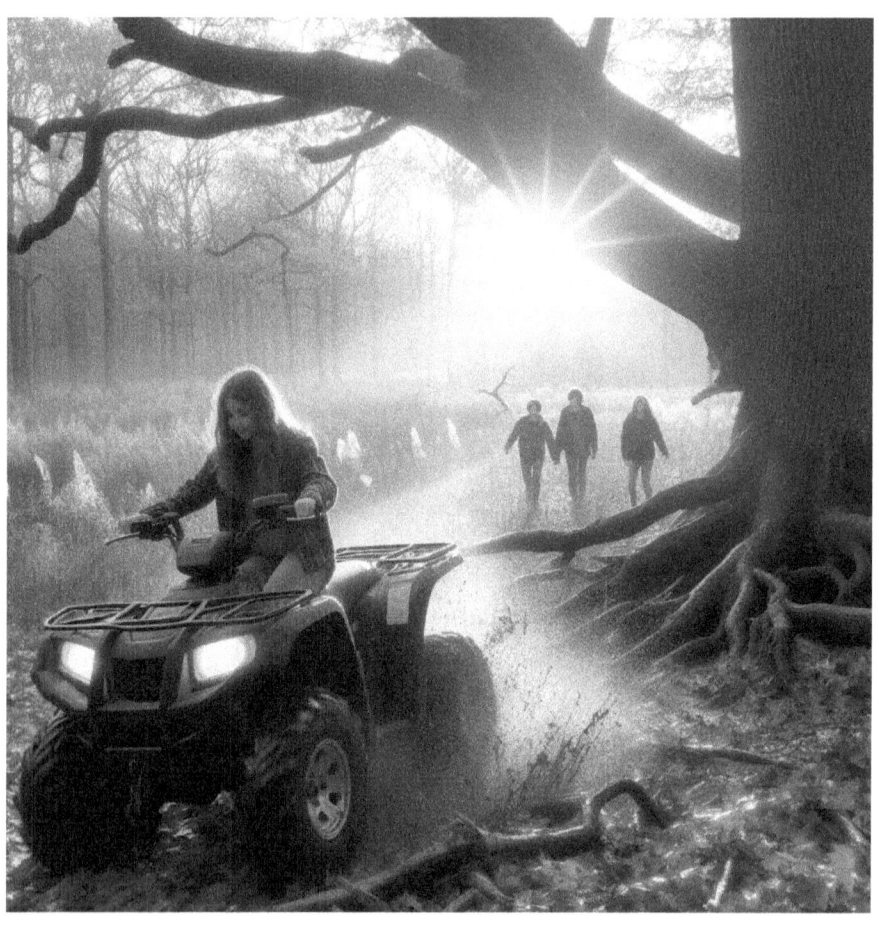

Samantha was thrown from the vehicle, her helmet striking the unforgiving trunk The world went black, her consciousness fading into the deafening silence of the forest. The sun-drenched afternoon, once a promise of adventure, now held the ominous shadow of tragedy.

Sarah and Mike, shaken but unharmed, scrambled to their feet. Panic surged through them as they saw Samantha lying motionless against the tree. Sarah's hands trembled as she fumbled for her phone, her voice quivering as she dialed 911. Mike knelt beside Samantha, his heart pounding in his chest, desperately calling her name, hoping for any sign of response.

The vibrant forest, once a playground of laughter, now stood as a silent witness to their fear and desperation.

The Emergency Medical Services (EMS) arrival was a whirlwind of activity. Assessing the severity of Samantha's head trauma, they called for a helicopter, the distinctive thrum of its rotors soon filling the air. Time blurred as the team worked to stabilize Samantha, securing her to a longboard, the urgency of her shallow breaths a stark counterpoint to the tranquil autumn day.

At the airbase, the crew's pagers erupted in a cacophony of alerts. The flight team received a pager message about a 14-year-old girl involved in an ATV accident with a head injury. Grabbing O-negative blood, they rushed to the helicopter, the familiar routine of pre-flight checks a comforting anchor amidst the uncertainty.

The flight was a tense dance of preparation and anticipation. The crew, seasoned professionals, knew the drill, yet each mission carried its unique weight. They discussed potential scenarios, their voices hushed against the roar of the engine, the sparse details of Samantha's condition fueling their concern.

Upon landing in a nearby field, the crew swiftly disembarked, their practiced movements belying the urgency of the situation. They entered the waiting ambulance, their eyes immediately drawn to the young girl lying motionless on the stretcher. Samantha's face, pale and still, bore the unmistakable marks of the accident. Her labored, shallow breaths painted a grim picture of her condition.

Dave, a seasoned flight nurse with years of experience, quickly assessed the situation and noted that Samantha's airway was compromised. Her breathing was insufficient to sustain her during the flight to the Trauma Center. A decision had to be made, and it had to be made quickly.

Intubation, a procedure to insert a breathing tube into the trachea, was the only viable option. It was a calculated risk, but the potential benefits far outweighed the risks. Dave, his hands steady despite the pressure, began the intricate process.

Samantha was sedated, her young body relaxing under the medication. Dave, with practiced precision, inserted a laryngoscope into Samantha's mouth, visualizing the vocal cords. A moment of tension hung in the air as he carefully guided the endotracheal tube into the trachea.

Once the tube was secured, Samantha's breathing was then supported and assisted by a ventilator. The rhythmic whooshing of the machine filled the cramped ambulance.

Dave's eyes scanned the monitors, his brow furrowed in concentration. Samantha's vital signs were stabilizing, the intubation a success. A collective sigh of relief swept through the crew, a momentary respite in the ongoing battle for Samantha's life.

The flight to the Level 1 Trauma Center was a blur of monitoring and silent prayers. Samantha's life hung in the balance, her fate entrusted to the skill of the crew and the resilience of her young body.

Shortly after taking Samantha to the Trauma Center, a computerized tomography (CT) scan was done which revealed diffuse axonal injury (DAI) – a severe type of traumatic brain injury resulting from sudden head velocity changes. DAI often leads to unconsciousness and a persistent vegetative state post severe head trauma, with a high percentage never regaining consciousness. Those who do wake up may face lasting cognitive and memory deficits.

The CT scan results painted a bleak picture for the girl's future. The crew left that day fearing she might never awaken. With Christmas approaching, it weighed heavily on them to think of the holidays ahead for Samantha and her family.

But then, a glimmer of hope emerged. Signs of improvement started to show, and within a week, the breathing tube was removed. Samantha not only recovered fully but also made it home in time for Christmas, a true miracle in the making.

The events that unfolded afterwards took an unexpected and heartwarming turn in the flight crew's lives. In a touching gesture, the mother of the Samantha contacted Dave and invited him to take part in a school project that her daughter, their patient, was actively engaged in. Dave accepted the invitation, and it wasn't long before he received an email from Samantha.

"I am Samantha XXXXX, you helped save my life, on November XX, 20XX when I was in an ATV accident. I am very thankful and would like to interview you for a school project, for Catholic Schools Week. A hero that made a difference in your life. Well, you helped save mine, so I have picked you. This project is due on January XX, so this Thursday I have volleyball practice, and Sunday I have a tournament. But any other day should be fine. If you have an available date please email or call my mom. I have returned to school and was cleared to go back to volleyball. I look forward to seeing you in the helicopter. Love, Samantha"

Dave and Samantha eventually met at the base where the flight crew had been working when they received the call. The sight of Samantha in such an ordinary state brought an overpowering feeling of joy. Samantha, the aircraft, and the team who helped her rescue were all captured in photos. Samantha and Dave spent close to an hour talking to each other.

A few days before Christmas, upon returning from a flight during one of their shifts, Dave discovered a small bag of holiday cookies and a Christmas card from Samantha and her family hanging on a doorknob. Realizing he played a minor role in this miraculous outcome remains one of the most heartwarming moments of his life.

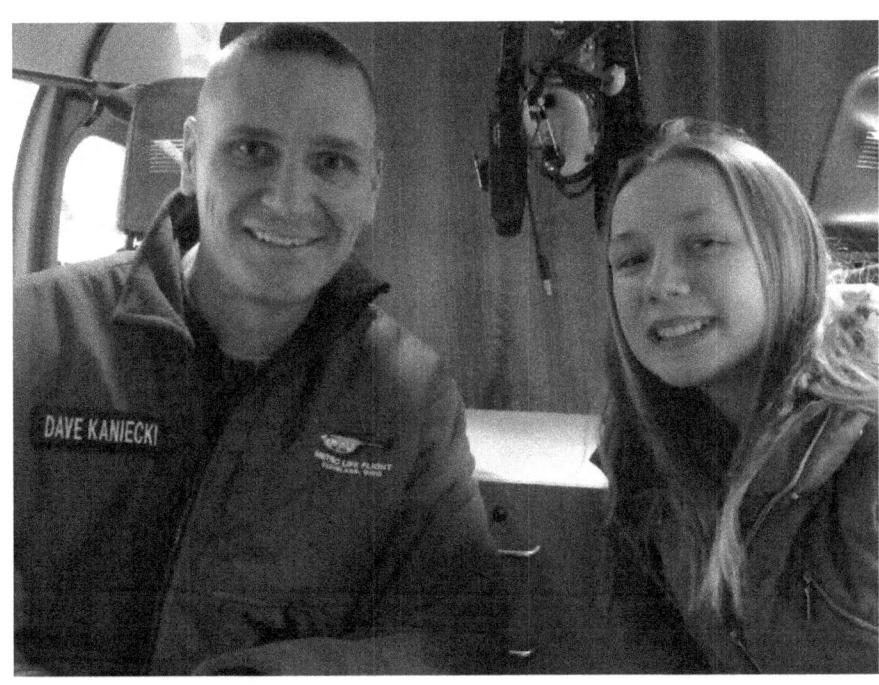

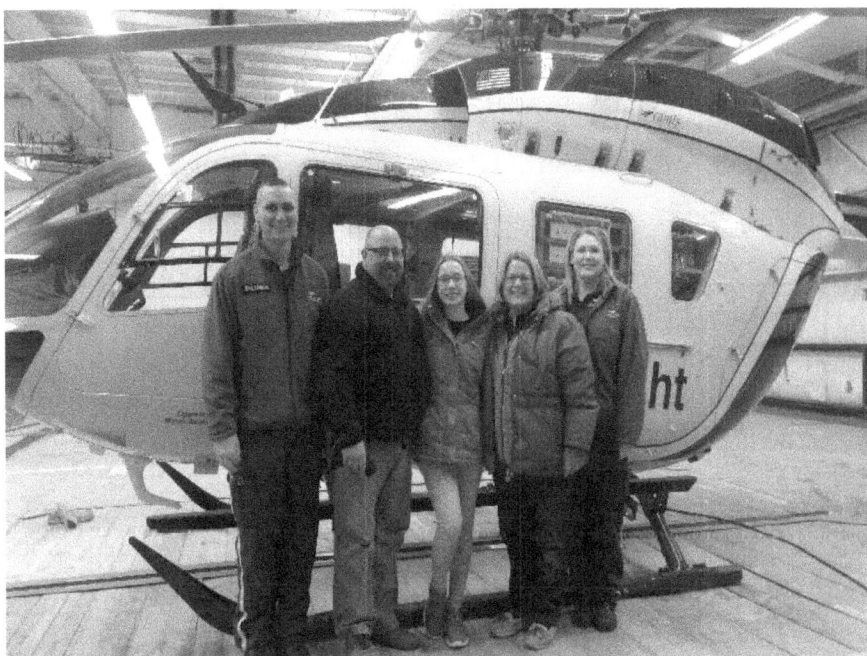

Engaging in activities like sports, cycling, motorcycling, ATV riding, horseback riding, or handling horses requires the use of properly fitted helmets tailored to each specific activity. These helmets not only save lives but also enhance neurological outcomes post-injury. The extensive body of evidence supporting their efficacy is compelling. Without a helmet, the outcome for the girl in this scenario would likely have been different.

Riding an All-Terrain Vehicle (ATV) can be an exhilarating experience, offering a unique way to explore off-road terrains. However, it can also be dangerous if proper precautions are not taken. Here's why riding an ATV can be hazardous and how you can make it safer:

Lack of protection: Unlike cars, ATVs lack a protective frame around the rider. This means in the event of a crash, the rider is more exposed to direct impacts.

Instability: ATVs have a high center of gravity and can be unstable on uneven surfaces. This can lead to rollovers, especially at high speeds or on steep inclines.

Inexperience: Many accidents occur due to riders not having adequate experience or training to handle the vehicle in challenging conditions.

Speeding: Excessive speed reduces the rider's reaction time and increases both the likelihood and severity of accidents.

Terrain hazards: Off-road terrains can be unpredictable with obstacles like rocks, tree roots, and ditches that can cause accidents.

Wear protective gear: Always wear a helmet, goggles, gloves, long sleeves, long pants, and over-the-ankle boots. Proper gear can significantly reduce the risk of serious injuries.

Get trained: Before riding, take a safety course to learn proper ATV handling and safety practices. Experience and knowledge can greatly enhance safety.

Inspect your ATV: Before each ride, check your ATV for any mechanical issues, including tire pressure, brakes, and fluid levels to ensure it's in good condition.

Ride at safe speeds: Adjust your speed to match the terrain and your skill level.

Stay on designated trails: Ride only on trails or areas designated for ATV use. These areas are chosen for their suitability and safety for riders.

Never ride impaired: Alcohol and drugs impair judgment and reaction times, increasing the risk of accidents. Never ride under the influence.

Ride according to your ability: Don't attempt maneuvers beyond your skill level or take risks that could lead to accidents.

Use appropriate ATVs: Ensure the ATV's size and power are appropriate for the rider's age and experience. Children, in particular, should not operate ATVs designed for adults.

By understanding the risks associated with ATV riding and taking proactive steps to mitigate these dangers, riders can enjoy a safer off-road experience.

A NEAR-FATAL OVERSIGHT

In the heart of a bustling city, a young mother named Jessica was preparing to drive her two-year-old daughter, Eliana, home from a birthday party. Laughter and the remnants of cake frosting lingered in the air as Jessica carried Eliana, drowsy and content, to the car. The evening was warm, and the promise of a cozy bed awaited them at home.

Jessica, having consumed a few glasses of wine at the party, felt a slight buzz but believed she was still capable of driving safely. She secured Eliana into her car seat, or so she thought, and fastened her own seatbelt. As they pulled away from the curb, the familiar route home seemed routine and uneventful.

However, as Jessica approached a busy intersection, her impaired judgment and slowed reflexes proved disastrous. Failing to notice a red light, she accelerated into the intersection, colliding with another vehicle that had the right of way. The impact was violent, and the sound of shattering glass and twisted metal filled the air.

In the backseat, Eliana, unrestrained due to her mother's oversight, was thrown forward with tremendous force. Her small body slammed into the front windshield, leaving a spiderweb of cracks and a trail of blood. The once-peaceful atmosphere was replaced by screams of pain and the frantic cries of onlookers.

Within minutes, sirens wailed as emergency responders arrived at the scene. Paramedics, working with practiced efficiency, carefully extricated Eliana from the wreckage. Her tiny body was limp, her face pale, and her breathing shallow. The severity of her injuries was immediately apparent.

Jessica, dazed and horrified by the realization of what she had done, watched helplessly as the paramedics worked to stabilize Eliana's condition. She knew in that moment that her selfish decision had nearly cost her daughter her life.

Realizing the need for specialized care, the paramedics called for a Life Flight helicopter to transport Eliana to a nearby children's hospital with a dedicated pediatric Trauma Center.

As the helicopter touched down in a field nearby, the medical team swiftly moved Eliana onto a stretcher and into the aircraft. Inside the cramped, noisy cabin, a seasoned flight nurse named Ethan took charge. The atmosphere was tense, filled with the rhythmic pulsing of the helicopter blades, the unending beeping of monitors, and the urgent chatter of the medical team. Ethan, nonetheless, stayed composed and concentrated, his years of experience guiding him through the crisis.

He carefully assessed Eliana, his expert eyes noting the severity of her injuries. Eliana's mental status was severely impaired, she appeared to have several broken bones, and possible internal bleeding. The force of the accident had caused a severe chest injury, leading to a collapsed lung. Ethan knew they were in a race against time. Recognizing the need for immediate intervention, Ethan instructed his team to start an IV line and administer fluids to combat shock and stabilize Eliana's blood pressure. He also administered pain medication to keep Eliana comfortable during the flight.

With the helicopter ascending, the city lights blurred beneath them. Ethan's mind raced, going over the steps he needed to take to keep Eliana alive. As the collapsed lung worsened, Eliana's breathing became increasingly affected, compelling him to act swiftly. To re-inflate Eliana's collapsed lung, Ethan would need to insert a chest tube.

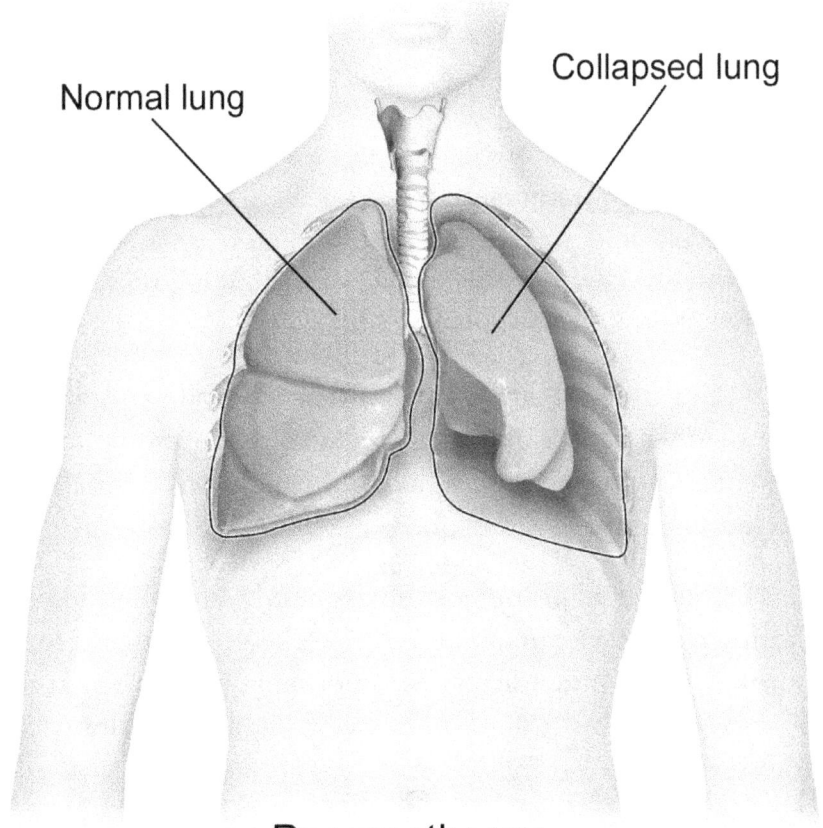

Pneumothorax

Ethan quickly prepared the necessary equipment, explaining the procedure to Eliana as best he could despite her condition and loud environment of the aircraft. He then made a small incision between Eliana's ribs, carefully inserting the chest tube into the pleural space surrounding the collapsed lung. The chest tube was connected to a drainage system, allowing air and fluid to escape from the pleural space, thereby re-inflating the lung.

With the chest tube in place and Eliana's lung re-inflated, Ethan turned his attention to her airway. Intubation, a procedure where a tube is inserted into the trachea to open the airway and assist with breathing, was necessary to ensure Eliana received enough oxygen.

Ethan skillfully intubated Eliana, carefully inserting the breathing tube and connecting it to a ventilator. He then adjusted the ventilator settings, closely monitoring Eliana's oxygen levels and adjusting the parameters as needed. The ventilator would breathe for Eliana, providing her with the vital oxygen her body desperately needed.

Ethan and his team worked efficiently and methodically, each movement precise and calculated. Inside the helicopter, the medical equipment cast a comforting glow, creating a restricted yet calming atmosphere.

Upon arrival at the hospital, Eliana was rushed into the operating room. A team of surgeons worked for hours to repair her broken bones and address her internal injuries. The surgery was successful, but Eliana's recovery would be long and arduous.

Jessica, filled with remorse and guilt, remained by her daughter's side throughout her hospitalization. She watched as

Eliana endured countless surgeries, painful physical therapy sessions, and the emotional trauma of the accident.

Over time, with the support of her family and a dedicated team of medical professionals, Eliana slowly regained her strength and spirit. Her physical injuries healed, and her emotional scars began to fade. Miraculously, Eliana made a full recovery, defying the odds and emerging from the ordeal stronger than ever.

Jessica's irresponsible actions did not go without legal repercussions. She was charged with driving under the influence, child endangerment, and reckless driving. The court, taking into account the severity of Eliana's injuries and Jessica's lack of prior offenses, sentenced her to a mandatory rehabilitation program, community service, and a suspended license.

Accepting her punishment, Jessica devoted her life to advocating against drunk driving. Hoping to prevent similar tragedies, she shared her story with others.

This heartbreaking story highlights the devastating consequences of driving while impaired. Even a small amount of alcohol can impair judgment, slow reflexes, and lead to life-altering decisions.

The consequences of impaired driving can be devastating. By making responsible choices and looking out for each other, we can significantly reduce the number of accidents and save lives. Here are some essential points to keep in mind:

Never drive under the influence: This includes alcohol, prescription medications, illegal drugs, or even over-the-counter medications that can cause drowsiness or impair judgment. If you're unsure, err on the side of caution and find an alternative way home.

Use a designated driver: When someone is intoxicated and needs a ride home, they can use ride-sharing services like Uber or Lyft, call a taxi, or take public transportation if available. Arranging for a designated driver or using community sober ride programs are also safe options. Additionally, reaching out to a trusted friend or family member for a ride can ensure they get home safely.

Child passenger safety: Children are particularly vulnerable in car accidents. Make sure they are always properly secured in a proper car seat or booster seat for their age and size. Double-check the straps are snug, the chest clip is at armpit level, and the seat is installed correctly according to the manufacturer's instructions.

Plan ahead: If you're going to be drinking, designate a sober driver before you head out. Alternatively, consider using public transportation, ride-sharing services, or calling a taxi.

Be a good friend: If you see someone who appears impaired, don't let them get behind the wheel. Offer them a ride, help them arrange a safe way home, or call a taxi for them.

Speak up: If you see someone who is about to drive drunk, don't hesitate to intervene. Talk to them, express your concern, and try to persuade them to find a safe alternative. If necessary, contact the authorities. Your actions could prevent a tragedy.

A SILENT THREAT

In a quaint suburban neighborhood, nestled amidst sprawling oak trees and manicured lawns, resided the Peterson family. Their home, a warm and inviting haven, was filled with the laughter of their two children, Amelia, a bright-eyed 8-year-old, and Ethan, her playful 5-year-old brother.

One chilly autumn evening, as the leaves outside transformed into a vibrant tapestry of red and gold, an unnoticed danger crept into their lives. The Peterson's aging furnace, tucked away in the basement, had developed a crack in its heat exchanger, silently releasing carbon monoxide into their home.

As the evening wore on, Amelia and Ethan began to complain of headaches and dizziness. Their parents, mistaking their symptoms for a common cold, offered them warm milk and tucked them into bed. Unbeknownst to them, the invisible and odorless gas was steadily poisoning their children.

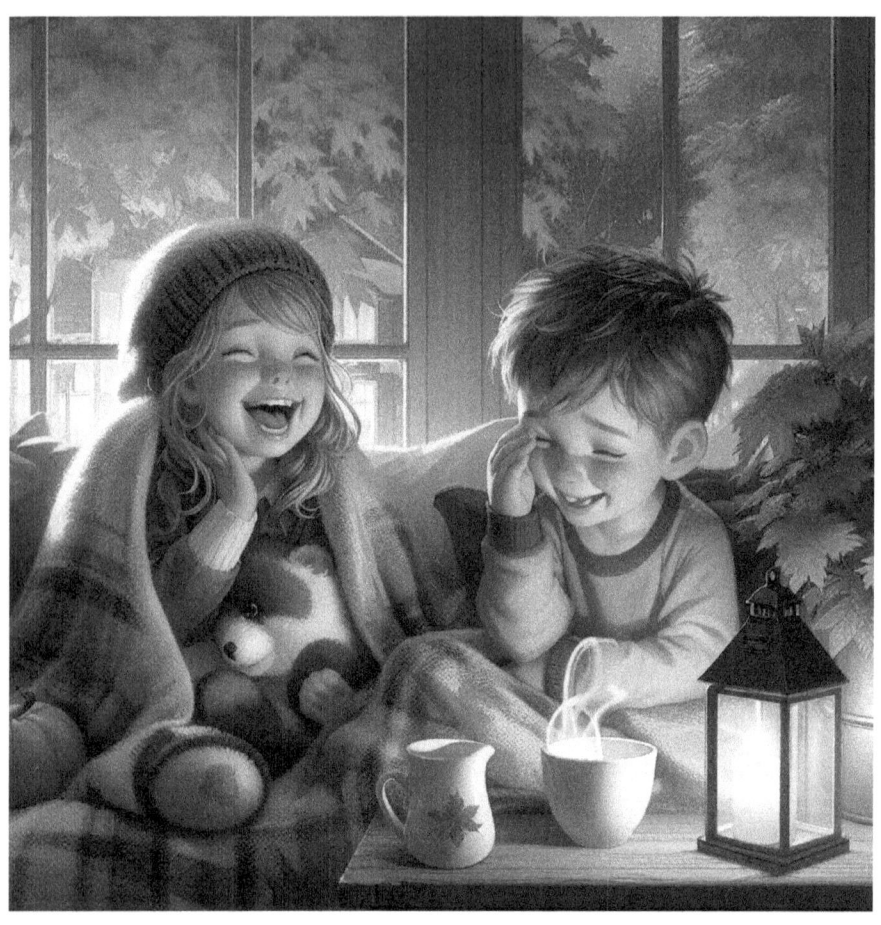

Hours later, Amelia's condition took a turn for the worse. She woke up feeling nauseous and disoriented, her breathing labored. Her parents, now alarmed and with headaches of their own, rushed her to the nearest hospital. Upon arrival, the medical team quickly recognized the signs of carbon monoxide poisoning.

Amelia was immediately placed on oxygen therapy, but her condition continued to deteriorate. The doctors, realizing the severity of the situation, decided to transfer her to a larger medical center with a specialized pediatric intensive care unit (PICU). However, the distance was too great for a ground ambulance, and time was of the essence. An air medical transport was requested, and soon the familiar sound of a helicopter's rotors filled the night sky.

The Life Flight crew, a well-coordinated team comprising a skilled pilot, a seasoned flight nurse named Sarah, and a dedicated flight paramedic named John, touched down on the hospital's helipad. Guided by security personnel, they swiftly made their way to the young patient, Amelia. Sarah, her expertise honed by years of critical care experience, immediately assessed Amelia's condition. The gravity of the situation was evident: Amelia's vital signs were unstable, her breathing was shallow and irregular, and her life hung in the balance.

In a race against time, the emergency department team, working in concert with the Life Flight crew, swiftly secured Amelia's airway by inserting a breathing tube to ensure adequate oxygenation. Once the tube's placement was confirmed, Amelia was placed on a ventilator, a mechanical lifeline that would breathe for her during the critical journey ahead. The team then carefully transferred Amelia into the helicopter, her fragile body entrusted to the skilled hands of Sarah and John.

The helicopter's interior, bathed in the soft glow of medical equipment, was a confined yet reassuring space. Sarah and John, with their movements precise and efficient, worked tirelessly as they administered medications, monitored vital signs, and provided constant vigilance to their young patient. The rhythmic thumping of the helicopter's rotors and the steady hum of medical equipment created a backdrop for their lifesaving efforts, a symphony of urgency and hope as they battled to stabilize Amelia's fragile condition.

Upon arrival at the larger medical center, Amelia was immediately taken to the PICU. A skilled and determined group of specialists labored tirelessly to ensure her survival.

The following days were a blur of tests, treatments, and anxious waiting for Amelia's parents. They stayed by her side, their hearts heavy with worry, praying for her recovery.

Slowly, Amelia's condition improved. With her vital signs stable and her breathing improving, the breathing tube was removed. She spent a couple of days in the PICU before being moved to a regular hospital room and then released the next day.

In the aftermath of Amelia's harrowing ordeal, the Peterson family, shaken to their core, resolved to transform their home into an impenetrable fortress against the silent threats of carbon monoxide and fire. Their journey towards enhanced safety began with a comprehensive evaluation of their home's vulnerabilities.

First and foremost, they installed carbon monoxide detectors on every level of their home, ensuring that no corner would be left unprotected. These vigilant sentinels, strategically placed near sleeping areas and in the basement, would sound an immediate alarm at the slightest hint of the deadly gas.

Next, they turned their attention to their aging furnace, the source of their recent nightmare. A certified HVAC technician conducted a thorough inspection, identifying and rectifying any potential issues. The cracked heat exchanger was replaced, and the entire system was meticulously cleaned and serviced to ensure optimal functioning.

Recognizing the importance of early fire detection, the Petersons installed smoke detectors in every bedroom, hallway, and common area. They opted for interconnected models, so that if one detector sensed smoke, all the detectors in the house would sound an alarm, providing precious seconds for escape.

The family also developed a comprehensive fire escape plan, mapping out two exits from every room and designating a safe meeting place outside. They practiced fire drills regularly, ensuring that everyone in the family knew what to do in case of an emergency.

In addition to these essential safety measures, the Petersons took proactive steps to eliminate fire hazards from their home. They decluttered their living spaces, removing any flammable materials that could fuel a fire. They also installed childproof covers on electrical outlets and kept cords out of reach to prevent accidental fires.

The Petersons' commitment to safety extended beyond their home. They educated themselves about fire prevention and carbon monoxide safety, sharing their knowledge with friends and neighbors. They became advocates for safety in their community, organizing workshops and awareness campaigns to help others protect their homes and loved ones.

Take Home Points

Here are some key takeaways from the story, emphasizing the importance of smoke and carbon monoxide alarms:

Silent danger: Carbon monoxide is an odorless, colorless, and tasteless gas, making it impossible to detect without specialized equipment. This story highlights the critical need for carbon monoxide detectors in every home.

Early detection: Early detection is crucial in preventing carbon monoxide poisoning. Symptoms like headaches, dizziness, nausea, and confusion can be easily mistaken for other illnesses, delaying treatment. Carbon monoxide detectors provide an early warning, allowing for prompt evacuation and medical attention.

Proper maintenance: Regular maintenance of heating systems, chimneys, and appliances is essential in preventing carbon monoxide leaks. The Petersons' aging furnace was the source of the leak, emphasizing the importance of inspections and repairs.

Timely response: In Amelia's case, the availability of air medical transport played a crucial role in her survival. It underscores the importance of access to specialized medical care in emergencies.

Family safety: The incident served as a wake-up call for the Petersons, highlighting the importance of prioritizing family safety. Installing carbon monoxide detectors, maintaining home appliances, and ensuring proper placement and regular testing of smoke detectors are simple steps that can prevent a tragedy.

Fire and Smoke Detector Safety Points

Proper placement: Install smoke detectors on every level of your home, inside each bedroom, and outside sleeping areas. Place them on the ceiling or high on the wall, away from air vents, windows, and ceiling fans.

Regular testing: Test smoke detectors monthly to ensure they are functioning correctly. Replace batteries at least once a year, or as recommended by the manufacturer.

Timely replacement: Smoke detectors should be replaced every 10 years, or sooner if they fail to respond to testing.

Interconnected alarms: Consider installing interconnected smoke detectors, so that when one alarm sounds, they all sound, providing an early warning throughout the home.

Fire escape plan: Develop a fire escape plan with two exits from every room and a designated meeting place outside. Practice the plan regularly with all family members.

CAMPFIRE CALAMITY

The sun dipped below the horizon, casting long shadows that stretched across the forest floor like gnarled fingers. A soft twilight descended upon the campsite, nestled deep within the embrace of towering pines and ancient oaks. The air was still and heavy with the scent of damp earth and wood smoke, a comforting aroma that spoke of wilderness and adventure.

A crackling campfire blazed at the heart of the clearing, its flames casting a warm, flickering glow that danced upon the faces of the campers gathered around. The fire pit, a circle of carefully arranged stones, held the fiery heart of the gathering, its edges licked by eager tongues of orange and yellow.

The campers, a group of friends seeking respite from the demands of everyday life, huddled close to the fire's warmth, their bodies casting elongated shadows that swayed and shifted with the flames' movements. Laughter and conversation flowed freely, punctuated by the occasional crackle of burning wood and the hooting of a distant owl.

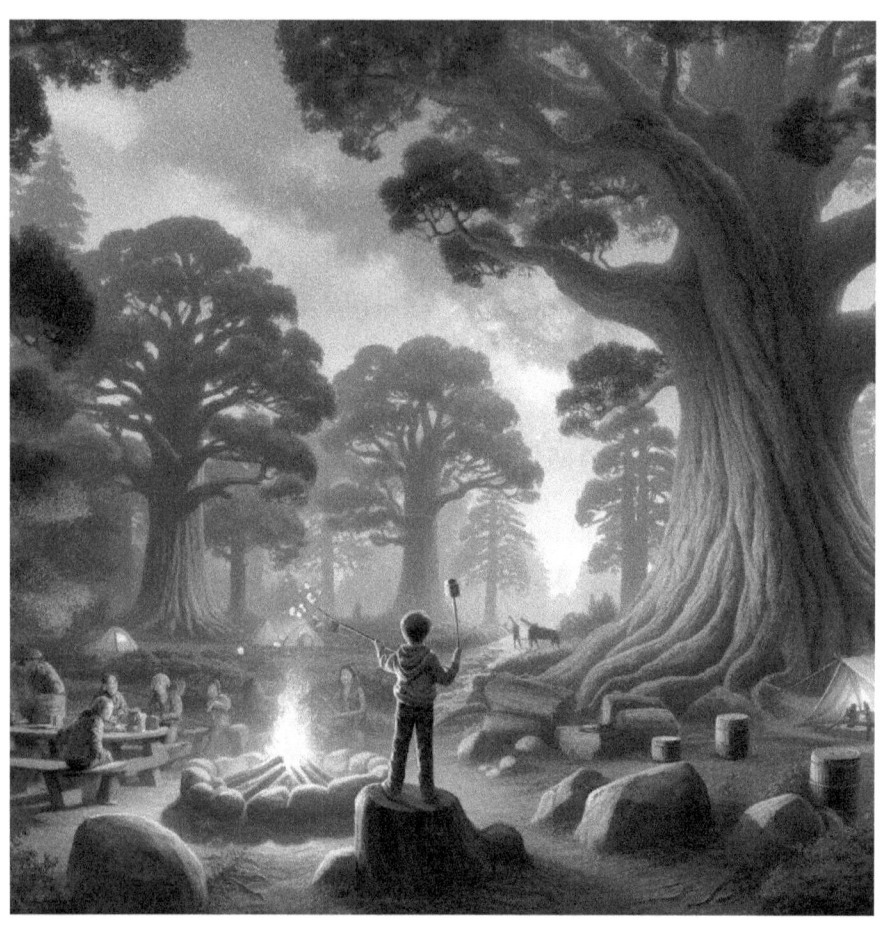

Among the campers was young Shawn, a spirited 8-year-old boy with an infectious grin and a boundless sense of curiosity. His eyes sparkled with excitement as he listened to the adults' stories, his imagination painting vivid pictures of daring exploits and hidden treasures.

As darkness deepened, the stars emerged one by one, twinkling like diamonds scattered across a velvet canopy. The Milky Way stretched across the sky, a shimmering river of light that seemed to flow into infinity. The scene was idyllic, a perfect tableau of camaraderie and contentment.

The adults decided it was time for the quintessential camping treat: roasted marshmallows. A bag of fluffy white confections was produced, and skewers were distributed to eager hands. Shawn, his eyes wide with anticipation, carefully threaded a marshmallow onto his skewer and held it over the flames.

The marshmallow began to toast, its surface turning a golden brown. Shawn, mesmerized by the transformation, leaned in closer, his face illuminated by the fire's glow. In his eagerness, he failed to notice the uneven ground beneath his feet.

Suddenly, his foot caught on a protruding root, and he stumbled forward. The skewer flew from his hand, and he pitched headlong into the fire pit. His screams pierced the night, a chilling counterpoint to the crackling flames.

The adults sprang into action, pulling Shawn from the fire and smothering the flames that clung to his clothes. His face was contorted in agony, his skin red and blistered. The severity of his injuries was immediately apparent.

Panic surged through the group as they realized the seriousness of the situation. The remote location of the campsite made it difficult to access immediate medical care. One of the adults, a quick-thinking individual, remembered seeing a ranger's station nearby. They grabbed a flashlight and sprinted towards the station, hoping to find help.

The ranger, a seasoned veteran of the wilderness, was shocked by the sight of the injured boy. He quickly assessed the situation, his calm and authoritative demeanor providing a much-needed sense of reassurance. The ranger carefully examined Shawn's burns, noting their severity and the potential for complications. He knew that time was of the essence and that Shawn needed specialized medical attention as soon as possible.

The ranger radioed for an air ambulance, providing details of Shawn's injuries and the campsite's remote location. He then turned his attention to providing first aid, drawing on his wilderness training and experience. He gently cleaned Shawn's wounds with a saline solution, applied a cool compress to reduce swelling, and covered the burns with sterile dressings.

Throughout the ordeal, the ranger spoke calmly and reassuringly to Shawn, explaining what he was doing and why. He offered words of comfort and encouragement, helping to alleviate the boy's fear and anxiety.

As they waited for the air ambulance, the ranger kept a close eye on Shawn's condition, monitoring his vital signs and checking for any signs of shock or infection. He knew that the next 30 minutes would be critical and that Shawn's life depended on the swift arrival of medical help.

The distant whirring of helicopter blades finally broke the silence, signaling the arrival of the Life Flight crew. The highly skilled team, consisting of a pilot, a flight nurse, and a paramedic, worked quickly and efficiently to assess Shawn's condition. They administered pain relief, carefully cleaned and dressed his burns, and prepared him for transport.

The flight nurse, Amanda, a compassionate woman with a gentle touch, held Shawn's hand and offered words of comfort, her calm demeanor a reassuring presence amidst the chaos. Shawn's mother, a pillar of strength despite her own fears, was allowed to accompany him on the flight, her presence providing an additional layer of comfort to her injured son.

The helicopter lifted off, its powerful rotors churning the air as it ascended into the night sky. The flight to the hospital was a blur of flashing lights and the steady hum of the engine.

162

Shawn, drifting in and out of consciousness, was vaguely aware of the sensation of movement and the muffled voices of the medical team working tirelessly to keep him stable. His mother, her hand tightly clasped in his, whispered words of love and encouragement, her voice a soothing balm to his troubled soul.

As the helicopter soared through the darkness, Amanda kept a watchful eye on Shawn's vital signs, monitoring his heart rate, blood pressure, and oxygen levels. She administered fluids to provide hydration and medication to manage his pain, her expertise and experience evident in every move. The paramedic, a skilled and experienced professional, assisted the flight nurse in providing care, his calm and steady presence a source of comfort to both Shawn and his mother. He adjusted the boy's dressings, ensuring they remained secure and sterile, and offered words of encouragement, reminding them that they were in good hands.

The flight, though seemingly endless, was in reality a testament to the efficiency and skill of the Life Flight crew. They navigated the darkness with precision, their expertise and training allowing them to provide critical care in a challenging environment. Shawn's mother, though filled with anxiety, was grateful for their expertise and the rapid transport they were providing.

Upon arrival at the hospital, the helicopter touched down on the rooftop helipad, its rotors slowing to a stop. The medical team sprang into action, transferring Shawn to a waiting gurney and rushing him into the emergency room, his mother following close behind.

The burn unit, a specialized team of doctors and nurses, was ready and waiting. They quickly assessed Shawn's injuries, their faces etched with concern. The burns were severe, covering a significant portion of his face and body, and requiring immediate medical attention.

Shawn was whisked away to the operating room, where a team of surgeons worked tirelessly to clean and debride his wounds, removing damaged tissue and applying skin grafts. The surgery was long and complex, but the skilled hands of the surgeons moved with precision and care. Shawn's mother, anxiously waiting outside the operating room, prayed for her son's strength and recovery.

In the days and weeks that followed, Shawn endured multiple surgeries and countless dressing changes, each one a painful ordeal. His face, once so full of life and laughter, was now a mask of scars. But Shawn's spirit remained unbroken. With the unwavering support of his family, especially his devoted mother, and the dedicated medical team, he faced each day with courage and determination. Slowly but surely, he began to heal, both physically and emotionally.

The incident left Shawn with facial scarring, a permanent reminder of the traumatic event. At first, Shawn was self-conscious about his appearance, feeling that his scars made him different and unattractive. However, with the support of his family and friends, he gradually learned to accept his scars as a part of his story, a testament to his survival and strength.

Take Home Points

When it comes to fire and campfire safety, vigilance is key. Always keep a watchful eye on children around any fire, ensuring they maintain a safe distance and understand the boundaries. Educate them on the "stop, drop, and roll" technique in case their clothing catches fire. Never leave a campfire unattended, and always have the tools to extinguish it at hand - a bucket of water or a shovel. Before leaving the area or retiring for the night, double-check that the fire is fully extinguished. These simple precautions can go a long way in preventing accidents and ensuring everyone's safety.

For immediate treatment of a burn, prioritize **halting the burning process:** if it's heat-related, remove the person from the source; if it's a chemical burn, remove any contaminated clothing and rinse with cool water. Next, **cool the burn** by running cool water over it for at least 10 minutes, or apply a cool compress if water isn't accessible. Quickly **remove any constricting** items like jewelry or tight clothing before swelling sets in. Afterwards, loosely **cover the burn** with a sterile bandage or clean cloth for protection.

Using ice or extremely cold water on a burn can make the injury worse by causing more harm to the tissues, similar to frostbite. This happens due to restricted blood flow, reducing oxygen and nutrients essential for healing. Consequently, this delays the healing process and increases the risk of infection. Additionally, the numbing effect of ice can mask the burn's severity, potentially delaying necessary treatment. It's crucial to use only cool water on burns and seek medical help if the burn is serious.

Over-the-counter pain medication can also be used for managing pain. Avoid breaking blisters, applying ointments, or using ice directly on the burn. Seek medical attention immediately for severe or extensive burns, those on sensitive areas, or if it's chemical or electrical in nature. Always remember, this is basic first aid; proper medical assessment and treatment are vital for any burn.

THE END

We should remember these children by learning from their experiences and using their stories as inspiration for action.

CREDITS

Cover Design: Haroon Ahmed

Reviewers: Laur Clark and Caroline Krauss

FOLLOW US ON FACEBOOK

To receive notifications of future publications, submit a story for potential publication, or share your experience with a life-flight rescue that others can learn from, please follow our Facebook page.

ABOUT THE AUTHOR

Dr. David M. Kaniecki, DNP, has an extensive background as an acute care nurse practitioner with expertise in emergency and critical care across both pre-hospital and in-patient environments. Dr. Kaniecki shares his expertise in books, industry journals, and formal academic instruction. By holding the position of faculty instructor and critical care transport education director at Case Western Reserve University, he plays a vital role in shaping the next generation of healthcare professionals.

Dr. Kaniecki is also the author of the book "Operation Flight Nurse: Real-Life Medical Emergencies." This publication aims to educate both the public and Emergency Medical Services (EMS) professionals about common medical emergencies and the critical interventions often necessary both pre-hospital and in the hospital setting.

Publications, Awards, and Innovations

Kaniecki, D. M. (2013). *Operation Flight Nurse: Real-Life Medical Emergencies.*

Kaniecki, D. M. (2024). Nurse Practitioners in Critical Care Transport. *Air Medical Journal.*

Kaniecki, D. M. (2019). Pericardiocentesis in an Ambulance: A Case Report and Lessons Learned. *Air Medical Journal.*

Kaniecki, D. M. (2017). Response of Flight Nurses in a Simulated Helicopter Environment. *Air Medical Journal.*

Kaniecki, D. M. (2013). Letter to the editors. Helicopter emergency. *Air Medical Journal.*

Reimer, A., Kaniecki, D., Ruszala, M., & Alfes, C. (2020). Usefulness of a Simulated Helicopter Transport Experience for Medical Resident Training. *Air Medical Journal.*

Cushing-Robb Scholarship for excellence in academic achievement, clinical nursing ability, and professional competence (2012).

Innovator Award – Cleveland Clinic Foundation (2012).

Conceptual device to reduce complications related to air embolism and hemodynamic monitoring. International Patent Application: PCT/US2012/054742 (2011).

www.ingramcontent.com/pod-product-compliance
Lightning Source LLC
Chambersburg PA
CBHW061751120626
46550CB00005B/1963